NURSE EDUCATION: a reflective approach

Edited by

Jan Reed
BA (Nursing), RGN, Dip Soc. Res PhD, Cert Ed

and

Susan Procter
RGN, BSc (Hons), PhD, Cert Ed
Institute of Health Sciences, University of Northumbria
at Newcastle, Newcastle upon Tyne

Edward Arnold
A member of the Hodder Headline Group
LONDON   MELBOURNE   AUCKLAND

Edward Arnold is a division of Hodder Headline PLC
338 Euston Road, London NW1 3BH

First published in the United Kingdom 1993

Whilst the advice and information in this book is believed to be true
and accurate at the date of going to press, neither the author nor the
publisher can accept any legal responsibility or liability for any errors
or omissions that may be made. In particular (but without limiting the
generality of the preceding disclaimer) every effort has been made to
check drug dosages; however, it is still possible that errors have
been missed. Furthermore, dosage schedules are constantly being
revised and new side effects recognised. For these reasons the reader
is strongly urged to consult the drug companies' printed instructions
before administering any of the drugs recommended in this book.

British Library Cataloguing in Publication Data
Reed, Jan
Nurse Education: A Reflective Approach
I. Title II. Procter, Susan
610.7307

ISBN 0-340-55786-9

10 9 8 7 6 5 4 3 2
99 98 97 96 95 94

Typeset in Times by Anneset
Printed and bound in the United Kingdom by
Athenaeum Press, Newcastle upon Tyne

NURSE EDUCATION:
a reflective approach

Preface

Over the past few years we have become very excited about some of the ideas being generated in nursing and education, namely ideas about reflective practice, mainly from Donald Schon, and ideas about expertise, Patricia Benner being the best known author in this area. As so often happens, we heard about these ideas through the grapevine – someone would mention them in conversation, an article would make reference to them, and so we decided to find out more. Finding out more was not as straightforward as we thought, however, as the texts were difficult to find, and we even had to resort to asking relatives visiting America to buy some of the texts, but eventually we succeeded.

When we started to look at these texts something struck us immediately. What these authors were saying was often quite different to the impressions we had gathered through the grapevine. This suggested that these ideas and terms were being used as clichés to pepper up conversations and articles, and the arguments that they were making were being distorted. This struck us as dangerous, for one of the central messages of this work was that nursing and education needed to debate these issues openly and freely, in order to break away from the old ideas of professional knowledge.

Nevertheless, the work that we read seemed to offer us some ideas about developing our courses. What had concerned us for a long time was the relationship of our teaching to our students' practice, and we had tried many ways to bridge this gap. Our mistake had been, we realised, that we had assumed our teaching was the only form of knowledge that was valid, and had therefore measured our success by the extent to which students analysed their work according to the theories that we had presented them with. We had not valued their knowledge or encouraged them to develop it, and if they could not apply theory to practice we had seen this as failure on the student's part, rather than on ours.

Reading Schon and Benner made us examine these assumptions more closely, and opened up a vast array of possibilities. The work was not, however, designed to be transplanted directly into a curriculum, or to provide a new set of procedures for teaching. Benner's work is simply an examination of expertise in practising nurses, and Schon's work does not directly address nursing, and so we had to distil some basic principles from this material, and adapt them to our situation.

At the same time, a number of changes were taking place in nurse education and in higher education. These involved new structures for both pre- and post-registration education, and we found ourselves being involved in these. The situation was chaotic in many ways, new ideas about knowledge, and new ideas about teaching combined to present us with a situation where everything was being questioned and debated, and nothing was sacred any more. Periods like this are very stressful, but also potentially very productive, in that they can allow innovation and experimentation previously unthought of.

This book is the equivalent of an interim report on our attempts at innovation and experimentation. What we have done so far is to develop a number of strategies and approaches, which are by no means perfect, and we expect to keep developing and refining our approaches continually. This development is based on continued debate amongst the staff, and so the book also contains chapters which outline these debates, albeit in a more coherent form!

We begin the book therefore, with a first section which deals with the background to changes in nurse education. Chapter One discusses the history of nurse education, highlighting the links between nursing and societal changes. This brings us up to the present day, and in particular looks at links between Colleges of Nursing and Midwifery and Higher Education, and the collaborative structures that this involves, such as conjoint validation, and joint course committees. Chapter Two examines nursing knowledge, looking at the different ways that this has been defined, and ending with a discussion of reflective practice. Chapter Three looks at the problems of developing reflective practice in nursing, problems which arise from the conflict of educational and clinical imperatives.

Sections Two, Three, and Four look at some of the approaches and strategies we have used in teaching. These strategies are not all about reflective education, as some deal with basic skills and knowledge, which we feel have to be taught in an abstract way but which we see as precursors to reflection. In order to reflect you need something to reflect with! This notion of different approaches for different types of learning can be illustrated by the following continuum:

Basic skills/ – Reflection
Knowledge
(Abstract and factual)   (Contextualised and discursive)
(Teacher as transmitter)   (Teacher as coach)
of knowledge)

At the basic knowledge end of the continuum (Section Two), the students need to understand the principles underpinning this type of knowledge, in a clear and thorough way. The amount of abstract discussion is therefore quite high, although learning can be facilitated by using examples of debates and situations which are drawn from the world of practice. The students cannot, however, derive this knowledge from practice nor, at first, can they evaluate or modify it. So the initial emphasis is on the acquisition of basic knowledge and skills. An example is Chapter Six which describes an Information technology package. This learning involves topics and concepts which are often unfamiliar to students, and requries some traditional learning of 'facts', before students can learn to use IT creatively. This does not means that this learning needs ot be done in a decontextualised way, however, and the chapter shows how students can be taught using examples of IT drawn from the world of clinical practice.

Some types of learning can combine learning basic knowledge with a greater emphasis on reflection; the examples given in Section Three are research methods and interpersonal communication skills. Here the links to the real world are much more vivid, communication is an issue which confronts practitioners daily, and research is becoming increasingly emphasised as a foundation for practice. The students are encouraged within the learning setting to debate and discuss the knowledge that they have gained – which includes not only knowledge from texts, but also experiential learning. Thus these strategies draw upon students' tacit knowledge of communication and research issues. All students will have some experience of communication, and (although they may not realise it) some experience of informal research, as they attempt, or see others attempt to find out more about practice. The emphasis is not on prescriptions for practice, but on using knowledge creatively and sensibly. This type of learning is somewhere in the middle of the continuum, as it involves the acquisition of knowledge, but also reflection on that knowledge. The teaching strategies in Section Three use a modified form of a *practicum*, described by Schon as an environment designed for learning which is not the real world but a *virtual* world. These practicums do not reflect all of the complexities of the practice world, but only focus on selected aspects of it. The emphasis throughout the teaching, however, is on drawing from practice experience to provide a context for learning.

At the Reflection end of the continuum, the focus is much more on the ways in which knowledge can be used in practice, rather than on the knowledge itself. Section Four deals with strategies which we have developed in order to facilitate this. Fundamental to these strategies is the explicit recognition of practice derived knowledge, and practice problems which demand creative thinking. The teaching strategies discussed in Section Four are critical incident workshops, clinical studies workbooks, and learning diaries. They all encourage students to reflect *on* practice using formal theory and theories-in-action. They do not represent reflection *in* practice – the analysis that students present is necessarily retrospective – but they do show students how reflection can be developed.

Section Five concludes the book. It deals with the thorny problem of assessment in Chapters Twelve and Thirteen, for we have found that assessing reflective practice is fraught with difficulty, and it is one of the perennial debates among staff and students. It is also a crucial issue, for if we wish practitioners to be reflective, then we must be able to identify and reward this in students. Chapter Fourteen links this debate to a discussion of the future possibilities for the development of nurse education, with a focus on post-registration education (one of the most pressing issues at the time of writing, as suggestions are made by professional bodies that advanced levels of practice should become formally recognised by the nursing profession). This notion is in many ways a long overdue development, but the debate about the form and nature of frameworks for such recognition is likely to be a long and complex one. Chapter Fourteen, therefore, gives an overview of these complexities, and examines the principles underlying the debates.

This book comes to few firm conclusions and is not intended as a 'blueprint' for nurse teachers; in fact, we would be very concerned if this became the case. Its purpose is to open up the debate about nurse education, to generate ideas, and to contribute towards a healthy, open, and collaborative discussion of where we should go next. It is likely that many others in nurse education have been involved in similar developments, and they may have had more success than we have had; if so, we would like to hear from them! The object of this book is not to claim that our way is the right way, but to begin to explore some of the ways that are open to us.

Newcastle upon Tyne   J.R.
April 1992   S.P.

Contents

List of Contributors

Joan Aarvold, Course leader for the Certificate in Information Technology course within the Institute. Joan is also responsible for teaching Information Technology and research appreciation to Project 2000 students at Newcastle and Northumbria College of Health Sciences.

Dr Brian Bell, Principal lecturer, involved in the development of Information Technology within the Institute, and in teaching on the Post-Graduate Diploma and MSc in Health and Social Research.

Joanne Bennett, Nurse tutor at Bede College of Nursing, responsible for community nursing components of pre-registration courses, and part of the BSc (Hons) Nursing Studies/RGN course team.

Steve Campbell was, at the time of writing this book, Senior Lecturer responsible for teaching Life Sciences on the BSc (Hons) Nursing Studies/RGN course within the Institute, and for teaching IT on a number of nursing courses. He is now a Lecturer in Nursing at Southampton University, and is chair of the Association of British Paediatric Nurses.

Dr Bob Heyman, Principal lecturer, course leader for the MSc in Health and Social research within the Institute, and head of the Research Division within the Institute.

Mike Kingham, Principal Lecturer, course leader for the Post-Graduate diploma in Health and Social Research, responsible for co-ordinating the teaching of sociology in the nursing courses throughout the Institute.

Jacqui Russell, Senior Education Manager (curriculum development) at Bede College of Nursing and Midwifery.

Anne Smith, Senior Education Manager at Bede college of Nursing and Midwifery and Course Leader for the BSc (Hons) Nursing Science/RGN/ course.

David O'Brien, Head of Division of Advanced Nursing within the Institute, responsible for curriculum planning and co-ordination.

Professor Don Watson, Head of the Institute of Health Sciences. A psychologist, he has extensive experience of CNAA committee membership and has been on a number of validation committees for nursing courses.

Graham Walton is Faculty Librarian (Social Sciences faculty) at the University of Northumbria at Newcastle. He was librarian for the Highland Health Board and then moved to Newcastle Polytechnic to set up a library and information service for trained nurses working within the Northern Regional Health Authority. His M.A. is in Educational Development, and he is currently chair of the Northern Regional Association of Health Service Librarians.

Section One
Nursing Practice, Knowledge and Education

Introduction

Before beginning to talk about teaching strategies it is important to debate the issues which lie behind them. Nurse education is not an end in itself, it is a means to an end, which is to develop skilled practitioners who can meet the health care needs of patients. Nurse education, therefore, is about nursing, and cannot be divorced from debates and issues in practice. This section seeks to give an overview of these debates, outlining the context in which nurse education is currently developing. The discussion begins with a historical overview of nurse education (Chapter One) in which the struggle for social respectability is described, followed by a discussion of nurses' attempts to consolidate this position and gain academic recognition. Chapter Two extends this debate by examining the development of nursing knowledge, posing the question 'Is academic respectability a useful route for nursing?' This question arises because of the limited usefulness and de-contextualised nature of traditional academic knowledge. Chapter Two concludes by identifying a possible way for academia and nursing to develop, by incorporating ideas of reflective practice into the types of knowledge regarded as valid.

Chapter Three, however, adds a note of caution. Reflective education cannot take place without a great deal of thought and care. It may also require changes in educational and practice structures. This chapter outlines some of the constraints that may confound the educator wishing to adopt the principles of reflective education, constraints which arise from the nature of nursing work and nursing organisation.

1 Nurse education: A social and historical perspective

David O'Brien and Don Watson

INTRODUCTION – THE SOCIAL CONTEXT OF NURSING CARE

Nurse education has undergone much change since the first training schools for nurses were opened in the last century. This change has been spasmodic rather than gradual, and it has been closely connected with corresponding changes in health care, societal values, and political concerns, both inside and outside the profession. Unfortunately, these factors have not always been pulling nurse education in the same direction at the same time – a situation which has made the overall direction of the profession uncertain, and caused many policies to seem contradictory. Response to social changes is appropriate for a profession which seeks to meet the needs of society, but it does reduce the ability of nursing to set its own agenda. We may feel now that nursing is in a position to determine its own priorities; the professional status of nursing is established, our expertise respected, and our autonomy guaranteed. This complacency could, however, be shaken at any moment. Nurse education is still, and always will be, subject to political and managerial decisions over which we may have little control, and the statutes which protect our status can be revoked. In these circumstances it is not surprising that our professional leaders have sought to consolidate and increase the social standing of nursing in the public eye. Public support makes a profession less vulnerable to political agendas, and more able to determine its own course.

Perhaps the entire history of nurse education can be seen as a striving for autonomy. In the beginning, when nursing first established itself as a legitimate occupation, the struggle was for social respectability, and the concerns of education were concerns about the conduct and morality of nurses. Having become accepted as a respectable occupation, we have now turned our attention to professional respectability, an equally difficult battle to fight. This professional respectability has become almost synonymous with academic respectability given that the criteria against which we judge ourselves are those derived from the systems existing in medicine, namely an undergraduate education. We are not necessarily aiming at a completely graduate profession but, in seeking to develop links with higher education, we are working to become part of the system that every other profession is part of.

THE ORIGINS OF NURSING AND MORAL EDUCATION

In 1848, as Florence Nightingale contemplated her vocation with people who were sick in hospital, many people would have been horrified, since hospitals:

> '. . . were places of wretchedness, degradation and squalor . . . gin and brandy were smuggled into the wards and fearful scenes took place . . . but their insuperable objection was the notorious morality of hospital nurses . . . it was practically unknown for a respectable woman to become a nurse.'

> (Woodham-Smith 1954).

Given this state of affairs it is hardly surprising that 12 years later, in 1860, with the inception of the 'Nightingale Systems of Nurse Education' at St. Thomas' Hospital, we find the conduct and character of would-be lady practitioners subject to considerable scrutiny. There was the implementation of a rigidly disciplined form of nurse training, accompanied by an emphasis upon hard uncomplaining service to patients. This suggests a perceived need to recruit a largely female workforce who would be 'self denying, hard working and amenable to discipline' (Davies 1986), if it were to be socially acceptable. In order to recruit women from 'respectable' backgrounds, nursing could not afford any suggestions that the moral education of trainees was in any way lacking. This approach not only became the predominately British way to train nurses, but it was exported to a galaxy of other nations.

The institution of such a system, in marked contrast to the previous employment of vagrants and drunkards, was made possible not only by the work of a number of individuals, but also by changes in social awareness of health care needs. The Crimean War had exposed serious gaps in welfare provision helped by the advent of mass (and relatively quick) forms of communication which had ensured that the British public were aware of the medical disasters being suffered by the Crimean troops during rather than after the campaign. The need for a nursing force to rival the French Sisters of Mercy became evident, although (as in nursing issues then and now) the doctors needed considerable persuasion as to the merits of the scheme.

The Nightingale notion of nurse education as essentially practical in nature, achievable with very limited resources, and informed by medical rather than nursing perspectives, was a notion suited to its time. Furthermore, given the status of women in Victorian society, it is difficult to see what other approach could have been used. It has however, left a legacy which subsequent nurses have tried to escape, and has arguably cast a shadow over all attempts to develop nursing autonomy since. Nightingale's notions of nurse education have meant that policy decisions during time of emergency (such as wars or during periods of demographic change when labour supply was scarce) have emphasised the need to recruit more nurses by decreasing entry requirements. The notion that nurse education is primarily concerned with ensuring a steady supply of conforming, obedient, non-critical young (mainly female) employees has become embedded in policy debates and has only recently been challenged. The perpetuation of such approaches to nurse education was dependent, however, upon a number of other factors.

Perhaps one of the most important factors was that of finance and economics. As the 19th century workhouses became, *de facto*, the first state hospitals (White 1984) and, with the growth of voluntary hospitals, the need to employ nurses began to grow causing concern for treasurers. The notion that nursing could be many things so long as it was cheap began to emerge with 'on the job' training being regarded as vastly preferable to any notion of systematic education.

The influence of the Nightingale Model of nurse education was extremely powerful and was supported by the prevailing social fabric. Within this culture the educational needs of women were given a low priority and women were generally subservient to men, thus the notion of a scantily educated nurse acting as the handmaiden to the doctor was easily sustainable. The result was a non threatening relationship between doctors and nurses with the doctor filling the instrumental, scientific clinical role and the nurse attending to the expressive, domestic and hygienic role. This role differentiation reflected gender role division in society and served to reinforce the prevailing attitudes to the training of nurses. Medical dominance meant that practice-relevant knowledge for nurses was deemed to be a pale reflection of that studied by doctors and that it was doctors rather than nurses who were involved in curriculum issues such as programme building (Jolley 1987).

Despite the enormity of the task, however, there were individuals who were prepared to voice their disapproval of this method of nurse training, and the idea that there should be state registration for nurses began to take shape. However, there were strong opponents to such registration (including Florence Nightingale) and even when, in 1919, the General Nursing Council (GNC) was established the war of attrition by the opposing camps had led to a Pyrrhic victory. The GNC was not the visionary body of nurse education with a well resourced Council able to make independent decisions in the service of nurse education. Instead, the GNC found its powers could be circumvented by government ministers, it had little direct authority in determining the nature and direction of nurse education and was even prevented from implementing a syllabus of training (Davies 1986).

The early promise of the GNC was, therefore, to be largely illusory. Nurse education remained subservient to service requirements, the movement from training to professional education was largely unattainable and nurses continued to receive their training 'on the job' with short periods of time in schools of nursing. In essence the past still held a powerful and pervasive influence over nurse education; tradition, ritual and unquestioning obedience tied nurse education to a previous era. This was reflected in the early training syllabuses and indeed in contemporary student nurse practice evaluation forms which still emphasise punctuality, smartness of dress and appropriate (subservient) professional behaviour.

PROFESSIONAL EDUCATION

Once again, however, the seeds of dissent were being sown. The Second World War saw significant social changes. Women were employed to undertake traditional male occupations and this brought greater emancipation. Following the Second World War educational opportunities for women began to expand and with this came wider occupational choice. Birth control and family planning meant that women could exercise biological control over childbirth which – combined with expanding social, educational and economic opportunities – resulted in a more liberated educated and independent female labour market. Such changes were in marked contrast to prevailing images of nursing which despite several government reports remained resistant to radical change.

During the 1960s and 1970s it was possible to detect changes which were to be the forerunners of the radical developments in nurse education being experienced today. Following the American tradition, a growing number of higher education institutions in the United Kingdom began to offer undergraduate nurse education and thereby set the scene for academic development within the profession. The search for a nursing body of knowledge as opposed to a medical model became established and by 1977 the GNC announced that the nursing process should become the prevailing philosophy for the organisation and delivery of nursing care. Nursing curricula began to emphasise socio-psychological aspects of care as well as patho-physiological dimensions combined with an emphasis upon problem solving and research utilisation.

The establishment of the United Kingdom Central Council for Nursing, Midwifery and Health Visiting (UKCC), and the four National Boards in 1979 quickened the pace of change. Curriculum development was quickly devolved to individual institutions rather than central control. Free to innovate, colleges of nursing developed a range of curricula and, by 1984, pre-Project 2000 pilot schemes had been introduced by the English National Board for Nursing Midwifery and Health Visiting (ENB). The contradictions and strains still remained, however, as the vast majority of student nurses still remained employees of Health Authorities and the tensions between educational and service demands were as acute as ever. Nurses were still largely trained in monotechnic schools or colleges and mainstream higher education influenced few student nurses.

It was against this backdrop in 1985 that the first working papers for Project 2000 were produced by the ENB with the final report in 1986. This report graphically highlighted the current context of nurse education and the need for change. In particular the report recognised how the status of the student is compromised by being expected to be at one and the same time, an employee of a Health Authority and a student. The report also discussed how nursing has become dependent upon high recruitment, high 'dropout' and poor retention of qualified nurses and the inevitable frustrations such an educational system causes for the student, the teacher, the manager and clinical colleagues.

The report further highlighted the changing world and the need for nurse education to be conscious of changing demographic trends in the population such as the growing percentage of the elderly in the population. The extent of chronic illness in contemporary society is also highlighted, together with the need for nursing to become more health orientated. This report suggests not only a change in the knowledge base of nursing, but also in the way that knowledge is developed, in other words that the pace of change in health care requires nurses who 'know how to learn', who are proficient in study skills, and who can keep pace with new developments

Among the major recommendations of the report was the need to restructure nurse registration courses to include a foundation studies and a branch programme, the need for supernumerary status for student nurses and the need for joint professional and academic validation with institutes of higher education (HE). These links with HE have the potential to further a professional agenda, in that nurse education will not remain marginalised at the fringes of academia, but will take a place within the system of HE of which most other professions are part. Becoming part of mainstream education allows nursing to argue the validity of its professional knowledge and status, and supports the argument that it has moved away from training (a non-professional system) to academic education. There is, however, some ambivalence towards this move, from nurses themselves and from some of the leaders of the profession. This ambivalence is perhaps due to anxieties about becoming part of a system which will 'take over' nursing, and will fail to recognise its particular concerns. Therefore becoming part of HE has been tempered with the insistence that educational and professional bodies are centrally involved with any developments.

The first of the six Project 2000 demonstration district courses commenced in January 1990 and an increasing number of students are now being recruited to an expanding number of such courses. This is also being paralleled by an increasing number of courses in centres of higher education leading to degrees and diplomas in nursing both at initial registration and at post-registration levels.

COLLABORATE LINKS WITH HIGHER EDUCATION

Project 2000 recommended that 'professional and academic validation should be pursued from the very outset of a process of change in order to achieve recognition of professional qualifications' (UKCC, 1986: p.59). The project group were aware that nursing qualifications generally had little or no academic recognition, primarily as a result of the non-student status of nursing students, and sought to redress this balance in the proposed Project 2000 courses. Links between nursing courses and centres of higher education had of course been well developed by courses in district nursing and health visiting and there were some, albeit limited, links between centres of higher education and colleges of nursing via undergraduate nursing courses.

However Project 2000 envisaged collaboration on a much wider scale with courses being conjointly validated (at diploma level) by the National Boards and the validating bodies of the centres of higher education. In essence this meant joint course planning and ultimately the movement of nurse education to a model more commensurate with higher education.

For the demonstration districts, the initial validations were surrounded by uncertainty and insecurity. The Royal College of Nursing recognised this problem in its Project 2000 briefing paper (RCN 1989) and while welcoming collaboration with higher education, expressed concerns about the location of nurse education, the nature of the teaching input and the optimum number of institutions of higher education to which colleges of nursing could link.

Such collaboration posed (and is still posing) considerable challenges for colleges of nursing and centres of higher education with new partnerships being formed as more Project 2000 courses commence. No single model of collaboration has emerged, though a popular one includes joint approaches to curriculum development and validation.

Higher education institutions – whether universities, polytechnics, or other colleges – have quite elaborate quality assurance mechanisms and procedures. New course have to proceed through a number of review stages before final validation and the commencement of the programme and, once validated, a number of monitoring procedures are required. Institutions vary in their approach to this exercise with polytechnics, through their association with the Council for National Academic Awards (CNAA), perhaps having a more detailed procedure. With the passing of the Further and Higher Education Bill by Parliament polytechnics now have university status, and the power to confer their own awards rather than those of the CNAA. One implication of this change, in addition to a proposed unified funding council, will be the establishment of a quality assessment unit for monitoring academic quality across the whole HE sector.

Currently, however, although practice varies slightly across HE, new proposed courses generally pass through a series (usually two or three) of internal stages, increasing in complexity and scrutiny before a final document is approved for the last stage of validation. 'Validation' is a rather generic term used to describe the process of academic quality assurance, and refers to the process or system of peer review whereby a judgement is reached by a group (which will include external assessors) as to whether a course designed to lead to a particular award meets the requirement for such an award. These requirements are determined by statutory principles and regulations which may be those of the particular university or, in the case of polytechnics, those of the CNAA.

More recently HE has entered into agreements with other accrediting agencies so that validation takes place in partnership. This process is referred to as 'Conjoint validation' and, in the case of Project 2000, the final validation of the course will be undertaken by a panel consisting of academic members of staff of the HE institution who are not nurses, external members with particular expertise in nurse education, and ENB members, including both Education Officers and elected members of the relevant ENB subject committees. The award is that of a Diploma in Higher Education with Registered Nurse (Dip HE/RN). The course team who present the proposal to the validation panel will usually comprise staff from the college of nursing who have designed the course, together with colleagues from the HE institution who are also members of the course planning team.

The documentation prepared by the team will address a variety of issues on which it can expect to be assessed by the validation panel, and which will have guided its planning. These issues will include both educational and resource issues as well as those relating to professional practice and statutory (ENB) regulations. Such issues are likely to include the following:

1. The validity and relevance of the structure and content of the programme, its coherence and progression, and the appropriateness of these for a Dip HE/RGN award.

Included within this issue would be related factors such as student selection mechanisms, how aims and objectives are realised, the intellectual demands made on the students, good professional practice, and the effectiveness and integration of the clinical/professional element.

2. The underlying philosophy and rationale of the course, and how this is translated into specific aims, objectives, and learning outcomes of the various stages of the programme.

Within this area the course team would be expected to demonstrate that the curriculum has been informed by current theory and approaches to nurse education, and that an appropriate educational model will facilitate such approaches.

3. The effectiveness of the approaches to the learning process and the teaching strategies employed to deliver the course.

This will include discussion of the appropriateness and balance of teaching and learning strategies in the proposed programme (which may take a variety of forms) and their relationship to aims, objectives, and assessment.

4. The appropriateness of assessment methods and the mechanisms for ensuring effective measurement of the performance of students, and how they relate to the teaching and learning strategies employed.

This will also involve discussion of the procedures for obtaining, evaluating, and acting upon student feedback and the regulations for passing and referring candidates at each stage of the course.

5. The resourcing of the course, including teaching and support staff, and the level and deployment of specialist facilities such as laboratories, information technology resources, and, most importantly, library provision and the appropriateness of the clinical learning environment.

6. The intellectual and professional quality of the teaching staff as demonstrated by scholarly and/or professional activity, including qualifications, research, contribution to the profession through published work, consultancy, conference papers, attendance on short courses, as set out in the Curriculum Vitae of individual members of staff.

There will also be discussion on the nature and form of the staff development programme and how this relates to the course.

7.   The mechanisms for quality assurance including the ability of the staff to monitor, critically evaluate, and maintain the standard of the programme.

This will include discussion of the delivery and management of the course and the effectiveness of the management structure proposed with reference to the formal responsibilities of the HE institution and the college of nursing, with respect to the programme and the students. There will also be some discussion of the contribution expected from external examiners for the course.

8.   Other general or institutional policies may also be relevant and need to be addressed during validation.

These could include such issues as equal opportunities, enterprise skills, modularisation, access, credit accumulation and transfer, and further educational/career opportunities.

In addition to the collaboration involved in the design and validation of the course, such models also usually involve joint representation on important committees, and where possible joint appointments and shared teaching and learning. Staff, for example, can expect to be members of committees such as the following.

1.   Examination boards

Although the college of nursing will be responsible for dealing with the statutory requirements for registration on a Dip HE/RGN course, the programme is 'jointly owned' by both parties, and the educational assessment of the students and the award of the Dip HE needs to accord with the HE institution's procedures. Examination boards, therefore, will consist of all staff providing a teaching input to the course and will be responsible to the HE institutions appropriate academic standards body or committee. Students on the Dip HE/RGN course thereby have the same rights of assessment and appeal as all other students in the HE institution.

2.   Course review committees

Although variously named, all higher education establishments will have some form of quality assurance system designed to monitor and keep under review its academic programmes. Courses may be required to submit annual reports on their 'general health', for example recruitment and retention rates, pass rates and student evaluation. Staff from both institutions involved may be members of such a review body or provide information to it.

3.   Other institutional committees.

Members of staff from either institution may also have cross representation on each other's standing committees, such as departmental boards, faculty boards, academic standards committees. The nature and extent of such membership may vary with the particular model of collaboration in place, but has the common purpose of furthering the links between the HE institution and the college of nursing (or colleges of health as some are now titled). This offers the potential to extend the nature of collaboration beyond the Project 2000 arena, to joint planning and co-operation in other programme areas, such as degrees in nursing, midwifery, or health studies.

In order to address these issues, and to agree finance and resourcing issues, several centres have devised a memorandum of co-operation which serves as a contract between the collaborating institutions stating the nature and functions of the proposed collaboration.

Less often, but perhaps more so in future, colleges of nursing have become departments or faculties of polytechnics or universities sometimes requiring geographic relocations. Obviously wholesale movement into higher education presents practical problems not just of physical location but the management of employees and their terms and conditions of service. Interestingly such a process was recently achieved in Australia and New Zealand, although it would be on a much larger scale in the United Kingdom given the greater numbers of HE institutions and colleges of nursing here.

The potential benefits of collaboration are considerable, involving accessing physical resources such as libraries, computing units and laboratories. Arguably, however, it is the possibility of staff collaboration which is the most exciting. A much wider pool of staff offers educational opportunities for students that have been unobtainable in the past. Teachers with specialist subject knowledge can offer new perspectives in curriculum development and nurse teacher colleagues from colleges of nursing can significantly expand and enhance the resource available to help service nursing and related courses in centres of higher education. One of the strengths of HE is that it can draw upon a wide range of experts in a number of different fields. This enables nurses to call in such staff for teaching purposes as and when necessary. This can be very flexible, as these staff have courses of their own to teach and are therefore ensured employment. When, or if, their input is no longer required, there is no problem of redundancy or redeployment as there would be if they worked exclusively for a college of nursing; and because they remain part of their own academic discipline, they can maintain up-to-date knowledge of developments in that discipline through daily contact with colleagues.

Perhaps more importantly, working in an multidisciplinary institution promotes the exchange of ideas between disciplines. For example, at Northumbria University we have a number of working groups discussing issues such as competencies or placement evaluation. These are concerns of nursing, but also of many other disciplines, and so these groups can be composed of nurses, engineers, chemists and librarians, to name but a few. In this way generic issues can be debated, problems compared, and experiences shared in what can be very fruitful discussions.

Another example of a concern shared by many disciplines is the need to develop 'reflective practitioners', that is professional practitioners who engage in continual evaluation of their professional practice through critical analysis, and who seek to develop, modify and extend theoretical understanding of practice and show how this informs and is informed by experience (Gallego and Walter 1991). This type of practitioner will clearly be more able to adapt to new knowledge and practice, and to be a more autonomous worker, as is recognised by many other disciplines apart from nursing. This development can be facilitated by discussions between members of different disciplines, who can distingiush between common and unique issues, and can learn from each other's experience. Such collaboration also provides the opportunity to develop the research base of nursing and since 'tomorrow's knowledge will be founded on today's research' (Birchenall 1991), the potential for developing the profession academically and professionally is considerable.

While the educational appeal of Project 2000, and the corresponding collaboration of higher education and colleges of nursing is very strong, there are undoubted problems – such as the very large size of many student groups, and the logistics of curriculum organisation. However, this might be the necessary price to pay for finally linking student nurse education to mainstream higher education.

CONCLUSION AND REVIEW

Contemporary approaches to nurse education in the United Kingdom have been powerfully influenced by social and political factors. Indeed, it might be argued that this educational debate within the profession has been secondary to these considerations.

In order to change the prevailing image of the nurse as a 'gin sodden' woman of ill repute, Florence Nightingale had not only to find a receptive society and supportive political system but had also to invest enormous emotional and personal energy. That she was successful in transforming the image of the nurse and nursing bears considerable testimony to her. However, paradoxically the inculcated value systems, the emotional fervour and the appeal to ritual and tradition created a nurse education system highly resistant to change.

During the past two decades, the 'driving force' for change has been gathering pace, albeit slowly and spasmodically. Changes in lifestyle, occupational expectations and educational opportunities, combined with demographic changes and changes in health expectations, have all served to quicken the pace of reform in nurse education. Having achieved social acceptability, in the sense that nursing is now considered to be a respectable occupation, the movement is now toward professional acceptability, in other words the acceptance of nursing as a self-directing profession. This move is linked with the acquisition of academic respectability, in that nursing is not content to remain a marginalised training system, but is seeking to become part of higher education.

This movement, however, has not been as straightforward as one might have hoped. Whereas the signing of collaborative agreements, and the forging of links between colleges of nursing and HE institutions may be a simple matter, there are a number of other issues to be considered. These involve not so much the suitability of nurse education to be part of HE, but the suitability of HE to be part of nurse education. These problems arise from the way knowledge in HE has been regarded, and its criteria for judging this knowledge, which are arguably esoteric, abstract, and not necessarily appropriate for practice. The next chapter discusses this problem in greater depth, comparing nursing practice with the traditional notions, still prevalent in HE, about valid knowledge.

REFERENCES

Birchenall, P.D. (1991) Preparing nurse teachers for their future role. *Nurse Education Today,* **11**, 100–2.

Davies, C. (1986) A constant casualty! Nurse education in Britain and the USA to 1939. In Davies, C. (ed.) *Rewriting Nursing History.* Croom Helm, London and Sydney.

English National Board for Nursing, Midwifery and Health Visiting (1990) *Framework for Continuing Professional Education and Training for Nurses, Midwives and Health Visitors.* ENB, London.

Gallego, A. and Walker, P. (1991) Preparation of health care teachers for the future. *Nurse Education Today,* **11**, 94–9.

Jolley, M. (1987) The weight of tradition; an historical examination of early educational and curriculum development. In Allan, P. and Jolley, M. (eds.) *The Curriculum in Nurse Education.* Croom Helm, London and Sydney.

Royal College of Nursing (1989) *What will happen to the Schools and Links with Further and Higher Education?* Project 2000 Briefing One. RCN, London.

United Kingdom Central Council for Nursing, Midwifery and Health Visiting (1986). *Project 2000* UKCC, London.

United Kingdom Central Council for Nursing, Midwifery and Health Visiting (1990) *The Report of the Post Registration Education and Practice Project.* UKCC, London.

White R. (1984). *Political Issues in Nursing: Past, Present and Future.* John Wiley & Sons, Chichester.

Woodham-Smith, C. (1954) *Florence Nightingale.* Constable, London.

2 Nursing knowledge: A critical examination

Jan Reed and Susan Procter

INTRODUCTION

The previous chapter has outlined some of the structural and policy changes in nurse education since nursing first emerged as a respectable occupation – changes which can be seen as a movement towards increased professional status. This movement makes the form and nature of nurse education a crucial debate for nursing, given that a central characteristic often cited of professional status is of a distinct body of knowledge, available only to those who have a recognised professional qualification.

If this definition is accepted, it then becomes necessary for any aspiring profession to identify, demarcate, and develop a body of knowledge, and to control access to it by means of an educational system. The educational system therefore bears a great deal of responsibility for professional development through its articulation of professional knowledge. In nursing this is a prime concern, for without the identification of nursing knowledge (as opposed to medical, sociological, or physiological knowledge for example) nurse education is no more than a watered down version of medical education, with fragments of the social sciences thrown in. Developing this body of knowledge is, however, problematic for a number of reasons. Firstly there is the nature of nursing work itself, in other words what nurses actually do, and how they do it. Despite several decades of nursing research, we still do not know a great deal about our work. This may be partly due to some of the features of nursing work; that it is seen as dirty, unskilled, and is therefore invisible, features which have not made it amenable to respectable scholarly study.

Secondly, there is the way which we have attempted to study nursing, and the way in which we have conceptualised theory and knowledge in nursing, in other words, our ideas of what is respectable scholarly study. In many ways this view appears to reflect the educational philosophies developed in ancient Greece, and in particular the work of Plato. Plato viewed abstract intellectual knowledge as a 'higher order' of knowledge than skilled (bodily) knowledge. Higher academic status was therefore attached to the ability to debate, at an esoteric level, the nature of 'good' or 'evil', or to produce definitions of abstract ideas such as 'beauty' or 'justice'. By contrast, skilled bodily knowledge – a nursing example would be how to lift a patient – which is dependent on the use of the senses and experience as well as knowledge, was regarded as low level everyday knowledge, unworthy of academic study.

It is clear that this distinction between intellectual knowledge and bodily skills remains a pervasive aspect of our education system, which systematically devalues psychomotor skills in favour of intellectual ability. Nursing falls directly into this schism, recognising as it does the importance of psychomotor skills, but being unable to grade such skills or accord them equal status with intellectual skills.

Both of these issues, the nature of nursing and the nature of knowledge form the basis of this chapter, issues which we feel are crucial to a debate on nurse education. It seems sensible to us to discuss the nature of the knowledge that we have, (or haven't) before we can discuss how to teach it. We start, therefore, by looking at some of the barriers to professionalism and developing a body of knowledge, problems which arise from the very nature of nursing itself.

NURSING WORK

Dirty work

Firstly, much of what nurses do is considered dirty and unmentionable in polite society. Nursing work involves dealing with faeces, vomit, urine, blood, and sputum, none of which, as Elias (1978) argues, have been the subject of social discussion since the 'civilising' of the body began in the 16th century. Hughes (1971), in his discussion of such dirty work, has described how, in the traditional Indian caste system, such work is relegated to the untouchables in society, and has argued that this is how societies deal with distasteful matters – by relegating them to those who are held in low esteem, and whose low status is reinforced by their work. Lawler (1991), in her study of how nurses deal with 'the problem of the body' described many interviews with nurses who reported that at social gatherings, disclosing their job often provoked a number of reactions, ranging from the horrified to the embarrassed. Even when people tried to respond positively, their approval was tinged with distaste, along the lines of 'I think you do a wonderful job, but I couldn't do that'. This type of backhanded compliment suggested to the nurses in the study that their perceived lack of fastidiousness marked them out as menial or somehow abnormal.

Given the association of nurses with the unmentionable and sordid aspects of human life (and this includes death, pain, and disfigurement in Western society) the claim of nursing to be a profession becomes hard to maintain. Interestingly, medicine does not appear to be tainted in the same way, although medical practitioners' contact with such matters is also frequent. Perhaps this is because the public image of doctors does not associate them as closely with the menial aspects of this work, a distance which is demonstrated in media portrayals of doctors and nurses, in which doctors will leave the cleaning up for the nurses. Peoples' own experiences of health care would also tend to reinforce this, as they are given evidence of the distasteful nature of nurses work, whereas the doctors' involvement with their body tends to be scientised and therefore sanitised.

Natural work

Paradoxically, the dirty work of nurses may be seen as abnormal, but also, in some contexts, natural. Some of the work that nurses do, particularly 'basic nursing' (a term that nurses sometimes themselves use) also occur outside nursing. The care of a mother for a baby, for example, and all the dirty work that entails, is seen as a natural, almost innate activity. Similarly, caring for an elderly relative is seen as demanding, but not requiring any particular skills or training. This lay caring (and there are probably more such carers than there are trained nurses in today's society) has been seen as so much the natural order of things, that it has until recently gone on without remark, and indeed many community care policies are based upon the assumption that this caring is unproblematic.

Nurses' attitudes to these lay carers are understandably ambivalent, as Lawler (1991) describes. At times nurses exclude them from care, particularly when the patient is in hospital, and Lawler suggests that this may have a protective function for the nurse, in that tasks can be performed without a critical audience, in addition to establishing and reinforcing the exclusive and specialised nature of their work with patients. In other situations, nurses can be seen to attempt to convert a supposed natural activity into one requiring education or training, as in parentcraft classes conducted by midwives and health visitors. These behaviours have the effect of distinguishing between lay carers and professional carers, by emphasising the body of knowledge and expertise that nurses have, which is a product of their education and training. Knowledge from training is established as more valuable than 'natural knowledge' – hence the need, for example, for mothers to be taught how to breast feed their babies.

Another way in which nurses have distinguished between lay and professional caring lies in the way that nurses have traditionally regarded the emotional component of caring. Lay carers may care because of their emotional commitment to the person being cared for, which may not necessarily be love, but may arise from their prior relationship with the patient. Nursing also claims a degree of commitment to those cared for, but this commitment is generally expressed as less personal and more abstract. Whereas a general commitment to the sick of society is laudable, this has been seen as only possible if nurses did not become 'over-involved' with individuals. In nursing courses, students have usually been warned against such over-involvement, in order to ensure their effective functioning as nurses (Benner 1984; Dunlop 1986).

This concern about over-involvement has some justification, in that it is difficult to imagine a nurse being able to cope with the daily tragedies of nursing without some degree of detachment. Being detached, however, also serves to distinguish between lay carers and nurses in the way that it emphasises the greater experience and 'scientific' approach that nurses have. Whereas a bereaved relative may have seen few people die, the nurse's detachment emphasises the normality of this occurrence in a profession which routinely deals with death.

Detachment may serve to differentiate between nurses and 'natural' (and therefore low status) caring, but it has not helped to differentiate between nurses and doctors. In attempting to achieve professional status, nurses have attempted to shed the 'doctor's handmaiden' image and develop an independent identity and set of values. Adhering to a detached approach becomes problematic in this attempt, as one of the central objections to the medical approach to health care, reflected in the nursing literature, has been the depersonalised approach of medicine, with its portrayal of patients as no more than their physical pathology. In order to be seen more than a subsidiary of medicine, nursing cannot adopt this approach.

This tension between the subjective and objective in nursing has been dealt with in a number of ways. Dunlop (1986) describes how, at an informal level, the nurse is exhorted to treat the patient 'as if' he or she were a loved one, a mechanism which draws upon the nurse's imaginative powers. Because it depends on imagination, however, distance is maintained – it recognises that this person is not actually a loved one, and that a conscious effort is required to treat such individuals as if they were. The 'as if' strategy is, however, a difficult one, demanding that the nurse walks a tightrope between closeness and distance which, Dunlop argues, 'always runs the risk of tipping either way'.

At a more formal level, nursing has attempted to address the emotional aspects of care by making these more central to discussions of the nurse's role. Although the giving of physical care has been used as a justification of nursing's claims to be a caring profession, the emphasis on the psychosocial can also be seen as an attempt to jettison this aspect in favour of 'cleaner' and more acceptable aspects. Dunlop has characterised this as 'the tendency to lose the bedpan' and describes the body as becoming more and more ethereal and marginalised in comparison with the emphasis on goals such as promoting psychological growth and meeting social and spiritual needs. By developing this emphasis, however, it can be argued that nursing is seeking to address the deficits of depersonalised care (the old strategy for creating distinctions between lay and professional carers), and creating a distinction on the basis of an informed and knowledgeable approach to the emotional. This separation of lay and professional caring serves to combat arguments that nursing is just a normal activity, and furthermore, one that is natural for females to perform.

Invisible work

The characteristics of nursing work, outlined above, serve to make nursing work invisible. Because it is 'dirty' it is not openly discussed or studied, and it is not publicly displayed. Because much of what nurses do involves aspects of living which are distasteful or even taboo, it is observed only by them and their patient. It is not amenable to media portrayal; whereas surgical operations have been televised in lurid detail, it is difficult to imagine a nurse giving an enema on peak television time!

Because much of nursing work is regarded as 'natural' or 'normal', it is invisible because it is not noticed. Much of nursing work is taken for granted, such as comforting gestures, or attendance to hygiene, and so has been largely ignored in research and discussion. Lawler, for example cites Elias's (1985) book 'The Loneliness of the Dying' which did not mention nurses or their care, an omission which can only be explained in terms of nursing work being so much taken for granted that it was invisible to the author.

The invisibility of nurses' work causes a number of problems in terms of nursing gaining professional status. Professional status comes, in part, from the acknowledgement in society that an occupation has a discrete body of knowledge, and furthermore that this knowledge is rational and 'scientific' i.e. it is based on research (Dickinson 1982). Invisible work makes the development of a body of knowledge problematic, should this be solely defined as based on research, given that research is a process which depends on making things visible, in order to analyse them. Many of the things nurses do are not observable to researchers unless nurses betray their ethical principles concerning the privacy of the patient. Even outside this private domain the things that nurses do may be, to the traditional detached observer, so normal and unremarkable that their significance cannot be appreciated or measured. The result of this invisibility is that we know very little, in a formal sense, of what nurses and patients really do, or why.

Nursing as skilled work

The nature of nursing work, that it is dirty, that it is natural, that it is invisible, can result in the notion that nursing can be regarded as an unskilled occupation, the chief requirements of which are a kind heart, and a willingness to work hard. This line of reasoning makes an increasing reliance on untrained, or minimally trained workers, a justifiable use of economic resources. Although there may be some acknowledgement of the need for trained nurses in a managerial or supervisory role, the need for trained nurses to deliver hands-on care is by no means universally supported either among nurses or to others outside nursing. Nursing has a long history of using untrained staff to give care, a situation which is accepted by many, in a way that reliance on untrained medical staff would not be (Dickinson 1982).

The argument against the reliance on untrained staff rests mainly on the strength of the ideological positions which nursing has developed, namely ideas of holistic and individualised care. It has been argued that these developments arose partly from a desire to scientise the emotional aspects of care, and make them amenable to rational discussion, and possibly also as a way of moving nursing away from dirty and menial work into the realms of psychology and sociology. There is, however, a strong altruistic motive behind these ideas, arising from an increasing awareness that depersonalised task allocation potentially created a great deal of distress in the recipients of care. Holistic care, which explicitly addresses the psycho-social aspects of living, and individualised care, which recognises the uniqueness of each patient, are both approaches to care which could potentially benefit the recipients of nursing care. In addition, they clearly require more from the nurse than a well-intentioned benevolence – they require a broad based education which includes knowledge from the life sciences and the social sciences.

Within this framework, the case for qualified staff becomes stronger. Holistic care, by definition, cannot be fragmented into tasks, and the use of unqualified workers would result in this (Procter 1989). As hospital stays become shorter, it is increasingly likely that patients will need technical care for a greater proportion of their stay, care which can only be given by qualified staff. To have this technical care given by nurses, and other care given by untrained staff would fragment care in a way unacceptable to those advocating holistic care. Similarly, as the importance of patient education and counselling becomes recognised, the trained nurse (who presumably has some insight into this area of patient care) cannot just be confined to this role while others give other types of care.

Interestingly, although the values of holistic and individualised care are presented as 'absolute values' which cannot be modified or diluted, there is evidence in the literature of attempts to reach a compromise between these humanistic ideologies and practicalities. One example is the research of Berry and Metcalfe (1986), which suggests that nurses do not adhere absolutely to particular approaches to care, but move between different approaches (the examples are task and patient allocation) as circumstances require. Even the prescriptive literature implies some room for manoeuvre. The literature on the nursing process which is a mechanism for organising holistic care, often distinguishes between planning care and giving it, suggesting that some adaptation is possible in the financially constrained health services, where care is often delegated to an unqualified workforce. Similarly the argument for nurse specialists, knowledgeable in only a specific domain of care, seems to suggest that it is not possible for nurses to be experts in all areas. A recent discussion of the nurse counsellor's role (Macleod Clark et al. 1991), for example, suggests that it is not possible for all nurses to have this degree of training or skill, and so this part of patient care can be passed on to an expert. This is clearly an attempt to reconcile the ideals of holistic patient care with the constraints that govern nursing practice, such as the shortage of training opportunities. In making this reconciliation, however, some ideals must be modified.

Despite these problems of implementation, the humanistic values of nursing provide the most coherent argument so far for the recognition of nursing as a skilled occupation, demanding a high level of education, and requiring investment in the development of its knowledge base. This development, however, is also problematic, given our ideas of what is respectable scholarly knowledge. The next section goes on to discuss these problems in greater depth, outlining the limitations of nursing science as it has been conceived and evaluated, and goes on to suggest a view of science which could overcome these problems

NURSING KNOWLEDGE

The central problem posed for nurse education by these humanistic ideologies, is their broad definition of nursing knowledge. Whereas in the past nurse education could concentrate on procedures and regulations, the demands of holistic care suggest that a nurse should be given a grounding in the life sciences, sociology, psychology, moral philosophy, social policy, and politics, to name but a few of the sources of nursing theory and concepts relevant to nursing.

None of these disciplines is distinctly nursing, but they all have a contribution to make. The question is, to what degree do nurses need to understand these disciplines in order to apply them? One view is the utilitarian one, that nurses should only learn what is directly applicable to patient care, and the measure of this knowledge is its usefulness. Another view, however, is that simply selecting fragments from a discipline divorces them from the context in which they were developed, and the debates of which they are part. The knowledge is therefore decontextualised and simplistic, and the critical abilities of the student are not developed. What emerges is a simple set of prescriptions for practice, akin to the old style of procedure-based knowledge.

The procedural approach is evident in many textbooks for nursing, where concepts from different disciplines are selectively and uncritically adapted to nursing practice. The reader, who has not had the advantage of a thorough understanding of these disciplines, is in no position to debate them. While this type of knowledge may meet the criteria of being easy to teach, it will not meet some of the other criteria of nurse education, namely that it should produce a critical, creative practitioner who has developed skills which will enable him or her to evaluate knowledge (and this includes new developments in knowledge), and apply it in a thoughtful way. This requirement applies not only to the contributory disciplines in nursing, but to nursing itself, whether this is seen as an amalgamation of other fields of knowledge, or whether it is seen as a unique body of knowledge in its own right.

The complexity of humanistic nursing presents problems for those wishing to define the knowledge base of the discipline, and so it is not surprising that there is a great deal of debate about how this should be done. For the purposes of describing this debate, we have divided the discussion into three different movements or 'camps'. There is the 'Academic Science' camp, whose members seek to develop nursing knowledge through the traditional scientific research approach, the 'Practice Knowledge' camp, which maintains that nursing is a practical occupation and as such should be learned through practice, and finally what we have called the 'Radical Academia' camp. This final movement is in some ways a blend of the others, in that it does use research, but it is radical in that it seeks to uncover practice knowledge rather than develop abstract theory.

Academic science

Advocates claim that it is only with an academic basis that nursing can become 'scientific'. This science is research based, full of 'hard facts', and as well as providing an 'objective' (rather than impressionistic) basis for nursing, also has a greater social value and status, and commands more respect than more subjective approaches to practice. The social value of academic education is well demonstrated by the medical profession, which is part of this tradition, and enjoys a higher status than nursing. Adherents of academic science cite support for their views from sources as diverse as

Florence Nightingale (1859) to the Briggs report (1972), and argue that without such science, theory and research, nursing will remain an unskilled and undervalued occupation.

This model of nursing knowledge presents relatively few problems for the nurse teacher, providing that he or she can gain access to, and understand, research and theory papers. In the classical technical rationality mode (Schon 1983), the knowledge base is developed by the academic elite, and the teacher simply transmits it to the students, who then put it into practice. Any problems that the students have in using this knowledge can be attributed to their lack of understanding (therefore the students need teaching in research appreciation) or the lack of understanding in the clinical staff (a similar remedy applies, but as this is likely to prove impossible, then we can only hope that these reactionary staff retire soon, or are inspired by the students to learn more).

Not surprisingly, however, this model of science has proved to be problematic, and has aroused protest from those who feel that it devalues practice-based knowledge. One such objection comes from those who argue that academic science, as it has traditionally been practised, is based upon the assumption that research is a superior form of knowledge which, because it is distanced from the phenomena it studies, is a 'better' form of knowledge. Writers such as Miller (1985) and Greenwood (1984) have argued that this assumption is flawed, and that this science produces irrelevant abstractions which cannot inform practice. Although academic activity may be intrinsically rewarding, and advantageous in career terms, it is essentially knowledge without responsibility or concern for those that it is meant to inform. This disinterested and aloof approach to science has a long tradition in other disciplines as Silverman (1985) describes, but whereas this may, at one time, have been felt valid in purely academic disciplines, it is questionable whether it is valid in a discipline which is very definitely applied, and moreover involves the care of vulnerable members of society, those who are receiving nursing care.

In addition to this problem of abstraction, this science is potentially at odds with the values of nursing. Webb (1984) has argued that academic science is patriarchal in that it assumes that the researcher or scientist's perspective is of more value than the research subject's. Hence researchers feel justified in controlling subjects, and withholding knowledge from them, in order to minimise 'contamination' of their findings. This approach is contrary to any principles of nursing which view the nurse-patient relationship as a partnership of equals, with different but equally valuable perspectives and knowledge.

Similarly, another criticism of academic science is that it is not in tune with the principles of holism in nursing. One approach to research and theory, namely the positivist approach, seeks to quantify and measure the social world in ways that are arguably incompatible with attempts to capture the totality of people and events. The argument is that measurement of limited aspects of care, which seeks to identify probable mechanisms of causality (at a statistically significant level) reduces people to a collection of variables and, although identifying general tendencies, cannot incorporate the variations between individuals and overlooks multiple causality.

These criticisms are, perhaps, applicable mainly to a positivist tradition of research and theory, and developments in qualitative approaches, action research, and grounded theory may go some way towards refuting the criticism that academic science is largely unrelated to practice. These approaches are not primarily concerned with making generalised statements about nursing, but with providing a detailed discussion of specific aspects and contexts of practice. Even these approaches, however, cannot guarantee findings of immediate and obvious relevance to nurses. This is not only because they too may involve abstract discussion, complex language, and methodological debates far removed from many nurses' worlds, but because no research can predict its findings. Research cannot always provide firm guidelines for practice, and indeed many would argue that research which tries to do this is in danger of finding easy answers at the expense of ignoring difficult questions.

Another aspect of academic science in nursing is the development of nursing models, which were envisaged as frameworks to guide nursing practice and education, and as starting points for the development of a 'universal' theory of nursing which would encompass all of the behaviours, issues, and contexts found in nursing. Part of their function is to delineate and define the remit of nursing, and therefore the required nursing knowledge. The theoretical status of these models is, however, dubious, some claiming only to be models (a fairly low position in the hierarchy of traditional theory development) and some describing themselves as theories (with connotations of rigor and predictive power, the criteria applied to traditional science).

Interestingly, nursing models, although allied to the academic science tradition, do not necessarily fulfil any of its criteria. They often have little or no research basis, and have not been empirically tested or validated. A number of writers, for example Greenwood (1984) and Hardy (1988), have argued that in fact they represent speculative or ethical statements of what nursing should be, rather than empirical statements about what nursing is. This changes, or should change, the debate to one about values and goals in nursing, rather than the academic respectability of the various theories. This debate is beginning to emerge, but it does more than critique models – it introduces a new way of developing nursing knowledge from a philosophical standpoint. This is an exciting development, and one which could generate great debate, but this is by no means guaranteed. As the understanding of philosophical methods tends to be limited in nursing, there is every chance that these complex arguments will be distilled into a simplified form, and disseminated as prescriptions for practice.

Perhaps the central problem of academic science is that it is developed by those in higher education (in fact by an elite group within higher education) and is therefore high status knowledge. The way of producing it is hidden to the rest of nursing, and so it is translated into prescriptions for practice. When academic science has a philosophical or ideological base, this problem is compounded, because not only is this science of high academic status, it also has high moral status, and so it becomes increasingly difficult to challenge. Those who question its relevance are also questioning its moral principles, and so become regarded as morally inadequate.

Practice knowledge

The discussion so far has suggested that theoretical academic nursing is fraught with a number of major problems, which limit its contribution to practice. What, then, are the alternatives? Advocates of practical approaches to education stress the values of the 'hands on' basis of developing skills. As much of nursing does demand manual skills, which are difficult to learn in a decontextualised way from a text-book or lecture, then the argument is that the best way to learn is from practice. Practice approaches are similar to the apprenticeship model of education, where skills are learnt from observation of others until the apprentice is able to carry out tasks unsupervised. Any theoretical basis is derived from practice, or from 'common sense', and although it may perpetuate custom and practice, it is at least realistic, and tailors practice to the circumstances in which it is carried out.

The perpetuation of custom and practice is, however, a central problem of practice based knowledge. As Friedson (1971) has argued, the professional's world is one which is 'prone to be self-validating and self-confirming'. This tendency arises because the professionals feel responsibility for the consequences of their actions, and therefore have no time to debate uncertainties, but must feel that their action is right or justified. Eraut (1985) also argues this point, using Mcluhan's notions of 'hot action', where there is no time for discussion because of the requirements for immediate action, as opposed to 'cold action' where there is time and opportunity to debate practice. Friedson also argues that the process of evaluation takes considerable time, but makes the additional point that 'it is psychologically stressful because it involves deskilling, risk, and information overload, when more and more gets treated as problematic while less and less gets taken for granted'. (Friedson 1971: p.128).

Where evaluation of practice is stressful, and resources for this evaluation are limited, the scene is set for the uncritical perpetuation of custom and practice, either personal or organisational. Theorists and researchers who identify this as a problem will not, however, improve the situation; they may only increase resistance to change or learning. What Eraut advocates, as a way out of this situation, is the creation of opportunities for professionals to 'escape' from their practice, so that they can reflect on it away from the demands of 'hot action', where responses have to be instant, demands are multiple, and there is no time for debate.

The issue is not just one of opportunity, however. If professionals are given time away from practice, this in itself will not produce thoughtful reflection, particularly if this time is spent on courses or study days in which they are told that they are incompetent or misguided, and that the solutions to their problems lie in textbooks. If, in addition, the practice knowledge that they have is dismissed and devalued (or perhaps not even acknowledged) then the results of such opportunities are likely to be unproductive. The problem is, perhaps, that clinical staff have not been able to articulate their knowledge in any way that has been viewed as academically respectable, and so the whole area of practice-based knowledge has been ignored or derided. This situation has changed, however, with academia now beginning to embrace and describe clinical expertise, a movement which we have termed, for the purposes of this book, 'radical academia'.

Radical academia

An example of this type of study, which seeks to uncover nursing knowledge in a way grounded in the everyday experience of nurses is provided by Lawler's (1991) work on 'somology', in other words how nurses deal with the problems of the body in nursing. Lawler describes the ways in which nurses skilfully manage the embarrassment of the patient when exposed in ways alien to everyday life, embarrassment which originates in the nature of the patient's dependence, where behaviours which are deemed private, such as defecation, have to be conducted with an audience of nurses. Interestingly, Lawler identifies a strategy used by nurses which involves a lack of observable reaction to the patient's behaviour at these times. This creates a climate of acceptance, in that the message conveyed to patients is that the nurse accepts the event as so routine that it does not even merit acknowledgement.

Strategies like this, which Lawler discovered, are used skilfully and selectively, are not the strategies recommended in most textbooks, if they mention such matters at all. In terms of research, these strategies could well be frowned upon by researchers who would code such behaviours as social conversation, or non-productive communication, as opposed to therapeutic communication. In many theories used in nursing, such lack of affect would be anathema to the warm, concerned, empathic approach advocated. Yet these strategies 'work', they meet the patients' needs, and they help nurses to cope with their job. The problem is that they are 'secret' strategies learnt in an informal way from colleagues, a process which can take time and result in inappropriate use.

Uncovering such secrets would seem to be a productive way to develop nursing knowledge in a relevant, realistic, and reflective way. It demands a re-thinking of research and theory, in that it requires an inductive approach to enquiry, and an emphasis on small-scale or mid-range theory, rather than the grand theories beloved of traditional science. Instead of attempting to explain nursing at a macro-level, an approach which involves simplification to the extent that the theory is 'as wide as an ocean and as deep as a puddle', perhaps nursing should concentrate on small-scale theories which acknowledge the differences and importance of practice contexts.

This 'radical academia' is also illustrated with reference to the work of Benner (1984). Benner's work vividly describes the decision making processes of expert nurses, and illustrates a level of practice which transcends the narrowness of research and personal opinion. These expert nurses have an almost intuitive grasp of situations which allows them to identify and prioritise needs, predict outcomes, and take effective action. In recognising and valuing this expertise, Benner has affirmed the value of practice knowledge, and made it more possible for others to articulate the basis of their practice and the rationales that they have for this practice.

Benner's work has a heuristic function for the whole profession, in that since her research it is now more possible for us to articulate our practice, and to listen to those who wish to relate their experiences.

Technical rationality and reflective practice

Radical academia may go some way towards reconciling the theorists and the practitioners in nursing, but there is also another issue to be addressed. This is not just about the type of knowledge a profession uses but concerns the way that knowledge is disseminated throughout a profession. This point can probably be best illustrated by reference to Schon's (1983) discussion of technical rationality.

Schon used the term 'technical rationality' to label theoretical knowledge developed in the reified environment of the university or research centre by a professional elite of researchers and theorists. This knowledge is abstract and generalised, and it is transmitted to the rest of the profession as a series of procedures or prescriptions for practice. Schon suggests, however, that while such knowledge can explain the world at a general level, it is inadequate in dealing with the everyday problems that practitioners meet in practice. He goes on to suggest that a good practitioner requires an extensive knowledge derived from technical rationality, but this in itself does not produce good practice. For good practice to ensue the practitioner must be able to select judiciously from the myriad theoretical perspectives they have learnt, those that are appropriate to the particular case with which they are confronted. Practice demands that knowledge and action are brought together – it is concerned with intervention. This is not a concern of science, which is concerned simply with explanation. Science therefore stops where practice starts.

For instance, if we take the example of a patient with breathing difficulties, knowledge of the respiratory system indicates that this patient should be nursed sitting upright as this facilitates expansion of the lungs. Knowledge of the circulatory system indicates that this patient may well have a reduced flow of oxygen to the skin which may increase his or her risk of developing pressure sores. Knowledge of the prevention of pressure sores indicates that the patient should be turned regularly to facilitate oxygenation of pressure points. The nurse caring for this patient has to decide the appropriate position for nursing him or her in order to minimise pressure on the sacral area without compromising an already reduced lung capacity. Essentially in solving one problem according to the dictates of technical rationality, you may well cause another.

It is this process of selection and rejection according to the specific and sometimes contradictory problems that patients present, which Schon suggests characterises everyday practice and distinguishes it from knowledge developed using technical rationality. This practice based knowledge, Schon argues, is a characteristic of the way in which professionals know about their world, a way which he called reflective practice. Reflective practice involves practitioners who can draw from a range of theories in a creative way, to address the particular, unique, and complex problems that they face in practice. They also begin to develop and create theories of their own, which Schon terms 'theories-in-action'.

Theories-in-action do not produce clear prescriptions for practice, and therefore one of the key aspects of this type of knowledge is uncertainty which, as Holden (1990) has argued, is uncomfortable for nurses. Uncertainty, however, is a normal feature of human life, and of all sciences which involve people (it is actually a feature of non-human sciences too, as chaos theory demonstrates). Denying or disguising this uncertainty may fit the traditional views of science as an attempt to predict and explain the world according to regularities, but it does not produce knowledge which is terribly useful, given that it over-simplifies the world. Reflective practice, on the other hand, is firmly linked to the 'messy' realities of practice; it is contextual and particular. It therefore is potentially more effective and more flexible than knowledge derived in the technical rationality mode. Using Schon's schema knowledge derived from this technical rationality moves from its position at the forefront of theoretical development to a more supportive role which underpins practice but is incapable of adequately explaining it. Schon does not dismiss academic knowledge entirely, in fact much of his research has focused on learning experiences which are dependent on the student's academic understanding of concepts, but his focus is on how these are modified and used in ways that are not simply procedural.

Similarly Eraut (1985) argues that a focus on the 'systematic' use of theory (a concept very similar to technical rationality) is a very limited focus; 'If we create expectations that theory is only used systematically, we direct attention from learning to use it in other ways and encourage its early dismissal as 'irrelevant' (Eraut 1985: p.123). This argument suggests that the real questions which confront practice are to do with the ways in which practitioners select, apply or reject theoretical perspectives during the course of their work in unique individual situations. According to Schon, a good practitioner is one who is skilled in the art of selection and rejection. Some practitioners, Schon claims, are much better at this process than others. He maintains their working practices should be studied in order to articulate the basis for their practice decisions and therefore make visible this process of selection and rejection – their reflective practice.

CONCLUSION

Schon's description of technical rationality is extremely relevant to past and current debates about the knowledge base of nursing, in that it corresponds very closely with the way in which nursing has attempted to define, develop, and implement nursing science. This nursing science has, until fairly recently, largely been associated with academic approaches to nursing, in contrast to the intuitive, 'subjective', and personal experience-based knowledge developed by practitioners, with the elevation of the former and the devaluation of the latter. 'Radical academia' can be seen as a challenge to this, since it explicitly seeks to uncover practice knowledge, and bring it into view.

Benner's work, and the work of other 'radical academics' could therefore make Schon's ideas about technical rationality redundant. This 'radical academia' is not the decontextualised theory that Schon critiques, and although still produced by an academic elite, its object is to give practitioners a voice, rather than drown them out. It could be argued therefore that Schon's ideas are based on what will be an increasingly out-dated idea of the relationship of theory and practice.

This argument is to a certain extent premature. The examination of practice knowledge is in its infancy, and much more work needs to be done before it can dethrone traditional academic endeavour. At present, this body of knowledge is an extremely delicate plant, and to burden it with the responsibility for changing existing views of practice and knowledge is to ask the impossible. In addition, any complacency about radical academia misses the central point of Schon's thesis, which is concerned with the way knowledge is disseminated and the way it is translated into rules and procedures for practitioners. There is no guarantee that practice knowledge will not become translated into new prescriptions for practice, just as decontextualised knowledge has been.

In some ways this is already happening. Benner's work in particular has been reified to form rigid criteria for expertise, and it will not be long before educational curricula and assessments are built around it. if indeed, this is not already happening. Once these ideas have become institutionalised it will become difficult to debate them openly in academic circles, and ironically, those practitioners who have misgivings may not be heard.

This does not mean that we must wait until vast amounts of literature have accumulated about practice knowledge before we can start to change our views of knowledge and education. Like Friedson's doctor, 'In emergencies [we] cannot wait for the discoveries of the future'. (Friedson 1971). What it does mean, however, is that we must be aware of the ever-present spectre of technical rationality, and conduct our debates with this in mind. This means that all those concerned in the debate must also have time away from the 'hot action' of argument; periods of reflection where they can think things through.

There is, however, an additional irony in the support given to the notion of reflective practice within nursing at the moment, and that is that reflective practice is in danger of becoming a mere slogan, with many using the words, but not necessarily thinking about their meaning or their implications. To return to the definition of reflective practice which we outlined earlier, this involves practitioners modifying and selecting theories in ways which fit their immediate practice problems. This may involve not only using theories in new ways, but also developing theories from practice and experience.

The reflective practitioner may therefore be a dangerous animal. Such practitioners' knowledge is not easily codifiable or communicable, and they are potentially disruptive in a profession which is seeking to define and demarcate its knowledge clearly. They will not necessarily adhere to procedures, and they may take risks, behaviour which makes them difficult to control or supervise, and which may make it difficult to ensure the legal safety of nurses and the physical and psychological safety of patients. In a profession which has a history of closely monitoring practice to ensure patient safety, the implications for our regulatory mechanisms may be considerable.

There are also implications for teaching. We cannot simply replace our old knowledge with the new knowledge, and teach it in the same way. We need to think about how we structure and organise learning experiences, so that yesterday's slogans do not simply become replaced by today's. We need to teach in ways which will encourage debate and reflection, which will help students to look at issues from a number of different perspectives, which will give them confidence in their own practice knowledge, and help them to evaluate and expand it. As Eraut (1985) argues, we need to extend our role from 'that of creator and transmitter of generalisable knowledge to that of enhancing the knowledge creation capacities of individuals and professional communities'.

This demands changes in the practice of teaching, in fact it demands that teachers reflect on their practice, draw from different theories, and develop their own theories-in-action. We cannot simply develop new systems or procedures for teaching, and crudely translate these into our practice, because everyone's practice will be different, and every problem we meet will be within a particular context.

There is another issue too. As we argued at the beginning of this chapter, nursing knowledge and therefore nurse education arises in its particular form because of the nature of nursing work. Developing reflective practice does not take away this context, and so nursing work must be taken into consideration when attempting this venture. This may seem obvious, as reflective practice is, by definition, linked with the realities of practice. Whereas other approaches, such as academic science, have attempted to deny or alter practice realities, this approach cannot do so. Having said this, however, there is no reason why the way that nursing work is organised should be fully compatible with educational imperatives, even if they are focused on practice issues. As the next chapter explores in more depth, the immediate concern of practice is patient care, whereas the immediate concern of education is student learning, and this can present a number of problems to those who wish to develop any educational framework, whatever this may be.

REFERENCES

Benner, P. (1984) *From Novice to Expert: Excellence and Power in Clinical Nursing*. Addison Wesley, California.

Berry, A.J. and Metcalfe, C.L. (1986) Paradigms and practices: the organisation and delivery of nursing care. *Journal of Advanced Nursing*, **11**, 589–97.

Briggs report (1972) *Report of the Committee on Nursing*. Cmnd 5115. HMSO, London.

Dickinson, S (1982) The Nursing Process and the professional status of nursing. *Nursing Times*, **78 (16)** 61–4.

Dunlop, M.J. (1986) Is a science of caring possible? *Journal of Advanced Nursing*, **11**, 661–70.

Elias, N. (1978) *The Civilising Process: The History of Manners*. Urizen Books, New York.
Elias, N. (1985) *The Loneliness of the Dying*. Basil Blackwell, Oxford.
Eraut, M. (1985) Knowledge creation and knowledge use in professional contexts. *Studies in Higher Education*. **10 (2)** 117–33.
Friedson, E (1971) *Profession of Medicine: A Study of the Sociology of Applied Knowledge*. Dodd Mead, New York.
Greenwood, J. (1984) Nursing research: a position paper. *Journal of Advanced Nursing* **9**, 77–?.
Hardy, L.K. (1988) Excellence in nursing through debate – the case of nursing theory. *Recent Advances in Nursing*, **21** 1-13.
Holden, R. (1990) Models, muddles, and medicine. *International Journal of Nursing Studies*, **27 (3)**, 223–234.
Hughes, E. (1971) Good people and dirty work. In *The Sociological Eye: Selected Papers*. Aldine Atherton, Chicago.
Lawler, J. (1991) *Behind the Screens. Nursing, Somology, and the problem of the Body*. Churchill Livingstone. Edinburgh.
Macleod Clark, J. Hopper, L. and Jesson, A. (1991) Communication skills – progression to counselling. *Nursing Times* **87(8)**, 41–43.
Miller, A. (1985) The relationship between nursing theory and nursing practice. *Journal of Advanced Nursing* **10**, 417–424.
Nightingale, F. (1859) *Notes on Nursing: What it is and what it is not*. Reprinted (1980) Churchill Livingstone, Edinburgh.
Procter, S. (1989) The functioning of nursing routines in the management of a transient workforce. *Journal of Advanced Nursing* **14**, 180–9.
Schon, D.A. (1983) *The Reflective Practitioner*. Temple Smith, London.
Silverman, D. (1985) *Qualitative Methodology and Sociology: Describing the Social World*. Gower Publishing, Aldershot.
Webb, C. (1984) Feminist methodology in nursing research. *Journal of Advanced Nursing* **9**, 249–50.

3 Teaching reflective practice: possibilities and constraints

Susan Procter and Jan Reed

INTRODUCTION

Reflective practice seems to be a positive direction for nursing practice and education to take. It offers the chance of developing knowledge which avoids the problems of academic science and also those of technical rationality, since reflective practice depends upon the critical and creative development of knowledge, which is linked to practice. Reflective practice, however, not only represents a change in practice, but also in education, and it is to this issue that we now turn. Changing our educational system is unlikely to be easy, and we cannot apply Schon's observations wholesale to the particular context of nursing. This chapter is therefore concerned with an examination of Schon's ideas, and a discussion of the issues that arise if they are to be used as a basis for nurse education.

COACHES AND PRACTICUMS

Schon (1987) suggests a number of differences between traditional educational styles and facilitating reflective practice. One of the central issues is the role of the teacher who will become, in Schon's schema, a coach rather than a transmitter of knowledge. On first examination, this coaching implies an androgogical perspective, treating the student as an independent adult with a capacity for self-directed learning. It also implies, however, a degree of expertise in the teacher, and an ability to articulate his or her mode of reflective practice in a way that is understandable to the student. The expertise of the teacher is clearly greater than that of the student, and confers on the teacher the duty and right to structure the student's learning experience. Students, almost by definition, cannot determine their own learning, because they do not know what they need to know, and therefore their learning must be guided. This suggests that although learning can be student-centred, in the sense that it focuses on the student's learning needs, it cannot be wholly student-directed. This does not completely rule out androgogy, as the coach can acknowledge the students' adulthood; indeed this acknowledgement underpins the learning process, for student nurses must function in an adult and responsible way as practitioners, but in order for this to be possible, the teacher must control and structure their learning.

This issue of teacher control can be illustrated by examining Schon's discussion of the learning environment as a *practicum*. By examining 'deviant traditions' in education, for example a design studio, Schon identifies a particular environment which he calls a 'practicum' . . . 'a setting designed for the task of learning a practice'. Schon goes onto explain that a practicum is '. . . a virtual world. It seeks to represent essential features of a practice to be learned while enabling students to experiment at low risk, vary the pace and focus of work, and go back to do things over when it seems useful to do so' (Schon 1987: p.170).

The concept of a virtual world, one that mirrors reality, but is in fact a protected environment, is very important in Schon's discussion of how teachers can manage the development of reflective practice. The need for the practicum, or virtual world, arises from the difficulties encountered by professional educators, across a range of disciplines, in integrating theory and practice. This cannot be left to chance, and so part of the coaching function is to develop and create practicums in which this integration can be developed. The onus is therefore on the teacher to control, structure, and order these environments, using his or her expert knowledge of real-life problems. This role is not necessarily congruent with simple student-centred approaches, demanding as it does that the teacher sets the agenda for learning.

According to Schon (1987), a practicum provides a learning environment that is designed to enable students to put into practice the theoretical knowledge they have already learnt. The aim of the practicum is to extend the students' understanding of theoretical knowledge by testing it out in environments which simulate the real world. Students discover both the insights that theoretical knowledge can give to an understanding of a situation and the limitations of this knowledge in solving concrete problems thrown up by the realities of practice. Students also learn how to blend theoretical perspectives and adapt them in a meaningful way to resolve the messy and contradictory problems presented by clients. This process of blending and adaptation of theoretical perspectives recognises that clients do not fit neatly into one framework and that each perspective probably offers some insights into the client's situation. The practitioner needs to be aware of all the different perspectives and the contribution they make to an understanding of a particular situation. But, over and above this, the practitioner needs to be able to decide how to prioritise between perspectives in order to determine a particular course of action.

A practicum, therefore, approximates the practice world, and in it students learn by doing in a way that is safe and supervised. Within the practicum students undertake projects and tasks, make decisions, and experiment with different approaches. Thus they can learn not only the ground rules and traditions of practice and forms of professional reasoning, but they can also devise new methods of reasoning – reflective practice.

The practicum, therefore, must have a number of key elements before it can develop the skills of reflective practice in students. Firstly, it must present students with the type of real-life problems and issues that they are likely to encounter in practice, with all their ambiguities and complexities. Faced with these messy problems, the students must also have a degree of freedom to make mistakes and choose unsuccessful strategies. In order to coach them through these processes of decision making, the students also need to have the presence of a teacher (or facilitator) in the practicum, who is able to present them with alternative frameworks they can try, enable them to discard and select information in a reflective way, and evaluate the outcome of their decisions.

The practicum, with the presence of a facilitator (rather than the traditional teacher who tells the students what to do), does not focus on traditional didactic methods of teaching. The emphasis is not so much on knowledge or 'facts' per se, but what students do with this information, i.e. not on what they learn, but on how they use the knowledge they have learnt. The practicum also extends the boundaries of knowledge, in that it focuses not just on the knowledge found in text-books, which is often idealised and decontextualised, but on the contexts and realities of the setting in which this knowledge will be used.

These principles have found support in nurse education, with nurse teachers experimenting with different methods and approaches such as contract learning and experiential learning, in order to facilitate the development of students as independent learners and practitioners. The arguments to support this move are very strong, arising not only from the limitations of traditional approaches with the resultant theory-practice gap, but also from an appreciation of the rapidly changing nature of nursing and health care. Nurse teachers have recognised that the traditional methods of knowledge acquisition, based on didactic teaching, may only equip students to meet the requirements of examinations and traditional assessments rather than enable them to relate their knowledge to practice. Nurses are increasingly being confronted with new knowledge, new structures, and new philosophies; there is therefore a strong argument for an education which will enable nurses to develop to meet these changes. This is an idea which has received increasing recognition in nursing over recent years, and it underpins developments such as Project 2000, the UKCC's post-registration proposals, and the ENB's concept of a Higher Award for nurses.

The ideal educational system then, to foster reflective practice, is characterised by the following elements: a problem solving focus based on the realities of practice, and coaching rather than instruction. These are possible within the practicum because it is an environment designed for learning, in which students can feel safe to practice and to learn from their mistakes. In the practicum they have the leisure and opportunity to analyse, critique, and evaluate their actions, and to experiment with different approaches in a safe but realistic setting. These freedoms exist because the practicum is not actually the real world, and because the students are encouraged to avail themselves of these opportunities by their teacher or coach. The teacher is there to give advice and suggestions, but also to challenge the students, acting as a role model through whom they can begin to understand the processes of reflective practice.

Practicums in pre-registration education

Developing the practicum in nurse education is, however, problematic. Whereas in architecture (one of the professions that Schon looked at) a virtual world can be created which does approximate the complexities of practice, in nursing this is much more difficult. This is due to the high level of complexity in nursing work arising from the interaction of different groups in an environment characterised by 'hot action'. In other words, a fundamental part of nursing is coping very quickly with multiple and conflicting demands in situations which can change rapidly. It may be possible to approximate this environment in the classroom, but what would be missing from it would be the sense of urgency which accompanies much nursing work. Whereas the practicum may give opportunities to reflect on practice, what happens within it will never present students with the same dilemmas as the real world.

The solution that immediately springs to mind is to use the real-life clinical environment as a practicum, a strategy which has become more possible since the introduction of the idea of supernumerary status for students. Traditionally within nurse education the clinical placements of student nurses have been regarded as the environment in which they can learn to apply theoretical knowledge to practice, in other words clinical placements operate as the practicum within nurse education. However there is a significant difference between a practicum as Schon describes it, and the clinical environment, and that is that the clinical environment is not 'a setting designed for the task of learning a practice', but it is a setting designed for the care of patients. In other words it is not a 'virtual world' but a 'real world'. While obvious, the implications of this fundamental difference have rarely been addressed in nurse education.

The fact that the clinical environment is a real world means that the extent to which student-centred learning can be upheld must be severely constrained and indeed subordinate to a patient's fundamental right to safe practice by a qualified practitioner. Most of the texts on student-centred learning emphasise the importance of allowing students to make their own decisions about how to solve problems. Intervention by the facilitator is limited to situations where help is asked for, or the student is obviously stuck and unable to progress. This is seen to give students the maximum control over their own learning, to reveal to the facilitator the level of understanding the student has of the problem and to teach students the process of problem solving within their chosen discipline. Within this framework, students are expected to make mistakes, which become a focus for further learning.

Clearly these principles can only operate within a virtual world. In a real world students can't learn by their mistakes, but must accept the decision of the qualified nurse even if they are not yet able to understand it. From an educational perspective this understanding could be developed if students were allowed to see what could go wrong if different decisions were taken. However, this would be untenable in a real situation – patients are not 'guinea pigs' for students to experiment with, especially since the consequences of making mistakes could be fatal. Therefore, within a clinical placement a much more didactic approach to student learning must be adopted. This reduces the opportunities for student-centred learning within the clinical environment but also recognises the important point, that education is a secondary rather than primary purpose of these settings.

The decisions taken by students in relation to patient care must therefore be mediated through a qualified practitioner and systems must be set up in the clinical placement to facilitate this. The setting up of these systems or procedures can, however, have a profound effect not only on the quality of student education, but also on the organisation of care on the ward.

Benner (1984), for example, found that even among qualified nurses, novices needed procedures as a means of entering the clinical environment. Procedures provide the method by which nurses can begin to practice nursing, without them they are lost. Procedures, therefore have an honourable role in nursing. Similarly Procter (1989) found that the care given on wards which depended heavily on student nurses as a major part of the workforce, tended to be dominated by routines. These routines were crucial as they enabled the qualified staff to manage the implementation of safe care via a transient and unknown workforce. Routines provided a safe system in which students could learn and care could be given. This suggests that not only may qualified staff affect students' practice, but the presence of students may affect the way in which the qualified staff work.

Part of the problem arises from the proportionately large number of students sent to each placement, compared with qualified staff, and the rapid turnover of these students. Taken together, this provides little opportunity for qualified staff to familiarise themselves with the particular learning needs of each student and to identify the student's current level of ability. This is particularly the case when qualified staff are also expected to assess and evaluate the care needs of each of their patients, which arguably should take priority over the needs of the student. Faced with these multiple demands and an unending flow of students, safe systems must be set up for dealing with the students in order to minimise the disruption to the unit which could arise if the educational needs of students were individually assessed. In fact the evidence appears to suggest that the extent to which routines or procedures dominate care is possibly related to the ratio of unqualified to qualified staff, the higher this ratio the more likely it is that care will be routinised (Benner 1984; Procter 1989). It is possible to argue that such a development is inevitable as it works in the interests of patient safety, and yet it directly contradicts many of the most cherished values of both nursing and nurse education. Moreover, the learning experience it provides is in direct opposition to the central tenet of much of the nursing curriculum, i.e. the value placed on individualised care.

It is, however, doubtful whether this problem can be overcome while there is a high throughput of students to the ward or community, who, as the curriculum grows, stay for shorter and shorter periods of time. Reducing the student numbers and increasing their length of stay on each ward would go some way to overcoming these problems. Increasing the time a student spends in each placement is extremely difficult as the curriculum tends to reflect the increasing specialisation in health care. In many ways this is embodied in the current EC regulations which specify the range of clinical placements to which a student must be allocated during training. Adhering to these regulations actually constrains attempts to promote stability in the training programme.

Supernumerary status and student learning

A major criticism of nurse education before the introduction of Project 2000 was the repetitive and in many ways routinised nature of the nursing experience of students within the clinical environment (Fretwell 1982; Orton 1981). Their role as workers as well as students meant that they spent much of their time meeting the basic care needs of patients. This care was seen by both the students and their educators as unskilled and lacking any educational potential. The introduction of supernumerary status offers the opportunity for students to participate, albeit under supervision, in the more technical and managerial aspects of care, which have been found to dominate much of the work of qualified staff. Thus it can be argued that this will provide a sounder educational basis for qualified practice.

There is, however, increasing evidence that it is during the implementation of basic nursing care that much of the hidden skills of nursing are learnt (Lawler 1991). A student-centred curriculum that enables students to identify their own learning needs is likely therefore to miss many of the important skills traditionally learnt by students during the course of their work with patients. As argued in the last chapter, however, our failure as a profession to acknowledge these skills or to identify them means that they frequently go unnoticed by the qualified staff, the nurse educators, and consequently by the students themselves.

There is, therefore, a central and unresolved problem in identifying what it is that students are expected to learn during clinical placements. This problem is exacerbated by the continuing tension between theory and practice in nursing and the frustration many nurse educators feel with the limitations which appear to characterise the educational experience of students during placement. It can be argued, however, that many of these limitations arise from the fact that the activities of students must be severely curtailed and controlled in situations where they are dealing with real patients. Ultimately it is the clinical staff that are accountable for the care received by patients, and clinical staff have to be satisfied that the care given falls within safe parameters.

It is possible to argue that the introduction of Project 2000 provides a means for overcoming many of the problems described above. Following its introduction students are supernumerary, ie. the ward staff are not dependent on them to give care. Their learning needs can therefore be identified and programmes instigated within the clinical environment to ensure that their needs are met. Even if this can be achieved, however, devising an appropriate programme of study may not fit easily into the clinical environment. According to Schon (1987), the role of the facilitator is to structure and organise the learning experience in such a way as to guide the student from a consideration of fairly simple problems to more complex ones as the student's mastery of the subject develops.

In nursing, however, some patients present with more complex problems than others; patients do not necessarily arrive in an order that facilitates the educational process. This means that students may encounter very complex situations before they encounter more straightforward cases. From this perspective the clinical placement cannot offer a graded exposure to the realities of practice. Instead, within the clinical environment students must confront the full complexity of patients' problems in their totality. Without careful planning and organisation of the learning experience this could be overwhelming for the student whose knowledge base and experience is inadequate for dealing with the situation.

It follows, therefore, that the clinical placement does not lend itself to student-directed learning and experimentation. Students cannot work at their own pace. The pace of work is dictated by external factors such as patient throughput, clinical decisions taken by medical staff which can radically alter the length and course of a patient's stay in hospital, as well as rapid changes in the patient's condition. By and large these factors are beyond the control of the nursing staff. While experienced qualified staff might be able to identify with reasonable certainty the duration and organisation of a patient's stay, this can never be ensured. Student projects which focus on the nursing care of a particular patient can be disrupted if that patient is summarily discharged, lodged in another ward because of pressure on beds, or referred or transferred to a different speciality.

Qualified staff as coaches in pre-registration education

Within this scenario the role of the mentor or facilitator is crucial in identifying a student's learning needs and devising an appropriate programme of study. But, while the students may be supernumerary, the mentors are not. This highly complex task is additional to their already crowded job description, a problem that frequently goes unacknowledged.

This conflict can be illustrated by looking at the example of a student who has been encouraged by a tutor to look at the health care given to a particular patient. This can be a very useful exercise, in the sense that this can help the student appreciate the complexity of holistic care. What happens, however, if the patient is transferred to another unit? One solution, facilitated by the advent of supernumerary status, is to allow the students to 'shadow' specific patients through the various medical specialities to which they are referred and even out into the community.

While supernumerary status makes such an innovation possible, the same cannot be said for a ward based facilitator or 'mentor', whose primary, and indeed full time occupation is to nurse the patients within a given ward or unit. If, in support of a holistic approach to care, nurse educationalists introduce a scheme of shadowing patients, it is possible that this will only increase the gap between the student's experience of practice and that of the qualified nurse, which is, or should be, the focus of training. It would appear that there is a mis-match between the current specialist and therefore fragmented structure of the Health Service and the ideals of holistic care which currently underpin many curriculum developments within nurse education.

The introduction of such a scheme, therefore, reduces the extent to which the mentor can facilitate student learning. It is not clear where the primary responsibility for teaching and guidance lies in such a scheme. It might be possible for nurse tutors to develop this role, however, the current staff:student ratios would probably prohibit this. In fact it is possible to argue that the costs of introducing a purely student centred curriculum in nursing which focuses on holistic practice in clinical placements are likely to be prohibitive, demanding as it does a 1:1 ratio in all placement-based learning situations. The alternative is a very fragmented learning situation in which the student shadows the patient through an increasing number of different departments and specialities. While this might enhance students' understanding of the need for a more holistic approach to patient care, they could make a similar plea in relation to their own educational experience.

It would appear, therefore, that for the foreseeable future qualified nurses working in clinical settings are going to continue to provide a substantive proportion of the education of student nurses. Given that students are training to become qualified nurses, such an arrangement seems sensible. However, as nurse educationalists know only too well, despite the best intentions, clinical placements frequently serve merely to exacerbate the theory-practice divide for each new generation of students.

It is possible to argue that part of the problem arises from the experiential knowledge or theories-in-use developed by ward or community based nurses which tend to reflect their own working experience of practice. In order to function effectively within the service, experienced nurse practitioners will need to develop theories-in-use which reflect the very fragmented and task orientated approach to care characterising the current organisation of the Health Service. Here task orientation refers to the task of the specialist unit within which the nurse works, for example medicine, surgery, psychiatry, theatres, out-patients, accident and emergency, intensive care, or specialist procedures such as dialysis or angiography. Even within the community such distinctions exist. The specialisation between community midwifery, health visiting, district nursing and community psychiatric nursing illustrates the problem.

This perhaps approaches the heart of the theory-practice divide in nursing. In developing a knowledge base for practice which derives not from experience but from abstract research, socio/psychological theories about the nature of man (for example Maslow 1970; Rogers 1951), and philosophical discourses about the definition of health and health care (for example Orem 1980; Roy 1980), the formal knowledge base of nursing has increasingly moved away from the concrete realities of practice. The theoretical frameworks subsequently produced are based on ethical arguments for holism and individualised care or from decontextualised research, both of which, it was argued in the previous chapter have high status, either moral or scientific. This makes challenging these theories very difficult, and possibly dangerous, in the sense that the challenger may be viewed as reactionary at best, and morally inadequate at worst.

The theories-in-use of practitioners are likely to be derived from and therefore to reflect the current organisation of care. In some cases they may perpetuate task-orientated and fragmented approaches to care as the most effective approach within the current structure of the Health Service. Within academic science such an approach has a priori been defined as 'bad practice'. For nurse practitioners to advocate their own theories-in-use as being more appropriate to the realities of nursing is by definition to advocate the perpetuation of 'bad practice'. To avoid accusations of bad practice, nurses must, therefore, espouse the academic theories.

This has the corollary that it simultaneously devalues the theories-in-use of practitioners, while promoting the 'enlightened' perspective produced by the academic science. This type of knowledge is rapidly incorporated into the nursing curriculum and taught to students who are sent out to the wards armed with a 'more enlightened' theoretical knowledge base than the qualified practitioners whose work they have come to study. Nursing abounds with tales of student nurses writing all the care plans following the introduction of the nursing process. Similarly, the sentiment is often expressed that learners 'keep the qualified staff on their toes' and 'make them keep up to date'. Practice without learners is seen as somehow stultifying.

The role of the student as the catalyst for the dissemination of new knowledge is taken for granted in nursing and yet from another perspective it is in many ways startling. If we return to Schon's definition of a practicum, the experienced practitioner is seen as the expert in dealing with the everyday realities of practice. Their theories-in-use, which enable them to function effectively within the practice environment, form a crucial knowledge base which cannot be captured by formal knowledge processes or taught within formal classroom settings. Reflective practice implies that if students are to become effective practitioners they must not only be exposed to practice-based knowledge, but learn how to use and develop it for themselves. In nursing, where the experiential knowledge of expert practitioners is systematically devalued, it can never be explored, analysed and learnt. The theory practice divide is, therefore, likely to continue in perpetuity.

Given this scenario, the aims and objectives of the clinical placement in nurse education become increasingly confused. Clearly, the experienced practitioner cannot be used as a facilitator to students, as he or she might teach theories-in-use which are useful in practice but conflict with academic science. As numerous research studies indicate students exist on a knife edge and learn very quickly which knowledge is used in which environment (see, for example, Melia 1987). While this indicates an ability for substantial reflection on their situation as student nurses, it does not help them to tackle effectively the complex problems of practice.

The role of the nurse tutor is equally ambiguous. Many tutors have experienced the conflicts that arise when trying to negotiate the introduction of new approaches to care in practice areas. Their understanding of the curriculum informs them that if wards don't introduce the changes advocated (e.g. use of the nursing process, adoption of a nursing model, or the practice of patient-centred care), then the ward may well be considered unsuitable for training. They have therefore to persuade ward staff to adopt the new knowledge.

Nurse tutors are not, however, in a position to test out these approaches in practice, neither can they modify them. In this situation, genuine difficulties identified by the ward staff can be re-interpreted as hostility to the changes proposed. Nurse tutors are frequently caught in the centre of this conflict. Often their own understanding of nursing informs them that the ward staff may have sound reasons for not adopting the changes in the format in which they are being presented, but their need to adhere to the curriculum means these arguments must be overcome. In neither case do the parties have the autonomy necessary to enter into genuine negotiations about the proposed changes and a stalemate situation is frequently encountered.

A way round this dilemma is, perhaps, to recognise and acknowledge openly the multiple perspectives found in nursing, in particular the traditional value systems which are found to dominate care giving in certain areas, and the progressive value systems which have evolved through the development of academic nursing. A major problem with nursing at an academic level has been an emphasis on unity and consensus in order to promote a coherent knowledge base. If, however, each perspective is seen as making a valuable contribution in its own right to the complex and messy problems thrown up by practice, then students could start to make judgements about which perspective is governing a given clinical situation and why. At a more advanced stage, they could start to analyse the situations they encounter in relation to the contribution traditional and new knowledge makes to a resolution of the problem presented. This develops a framework for students to reflect on practice and develop their critical faculties in relation to their chosen occupation and not according to a set of abstract academic principles.

Using this strategy, the views and knowledge of nurses who take a traditional approach to care become a valuable resource which students can use to gain greater insight into the complexities of nursing care. In this way the tacit knowledge and skills developed by experienced nurses are made available to students and not lost in the vanguard of idealism. Students could be encouraged to debate the different perspectives in the light of their clinical experience, and may sometimes conclude that the traditional approach is perhaps the most appropriate for resolving a given problem. Thus the theories- in-use of practising nurses are valued alongside the new knowledge as they provide a pragmatic and knowledgable response to the demands of practice. Students, in debating the contribution made by the different perspectives, could be expected to indicate an appreciation of traditional knowledge and the contribution it makes to patient care.

Coaches and practicums in post-registration education

These debates are also relevant to the post-registration education of qualified nurses. Their 'clinical placement' is usually where they work, or certainly where they are expected to perform as a qualified nurse. If the course is a clinical one, then their lack of expertise in that particular area is acknowledged, sometimes to a ridiculous extent (for example registered nurses doing some post-basic courses are not allowed to do certain tasks such as taking blood pressure readings, because they are 'students'). For courses such as the DPSN and part-time nursing degrees, the student is in a different position. At work they are fully functioning members of the workforce, and often quite senior. On the course they are academic novices, a situation which can lead them to doubt their clinical knowledge. This problem manifests itself in an over-respectful approach to literature, and a tendency to devalue the work that they do.

If the concern of the course is to develop reflective practice, then it must allow these students to recognise their expertise and knowledge, and coach them in describing and articulating it. The post-registration students' problem is not that 'they do not know what they need to know', more that 'they do not know what they *do* know'. This idea does not necessarily glorify the practitioner unduly; we are not claiming that by virtue of qualification and a period of practice, the nurse must automatically be considered an expert in the job, who requires little or no teaching, but it has to be recognised that the student knows, much better than the teacher, what the realities of practice are.

The basic aim of this type of post-registration course is to allow students to recognise and then develop this knowledge (Eraut 1985). Basic competence and safety can be assumed, and so in this sense the course can move beyond these issues more easily than a pre-registration course. There are, however, some problems which Project 2000 has attempted to address for pre-registration training, but which remain major issues in post-registration, namely the non- supernumary status of the student, and the lack of clinical mentors who can provide exemplars of reflective practice.

Where students are part of the workforce, their primary duty is inevitably to the employing organisation, rather than to the educational establishment. This can cause disruptions in attendance and course learning when work pressures increase. Teachers and students can become angry about this, seeing the employer or manager as unsupportive or destructive, and resenting the demands of work. This falls into the same trap as pre- registration education debates fall into, however, that of treating the world of patient care as one devoted to learning, whereas it is centred on patient care.

It is possible, as some of our students have shown, to use these situations as the basis for course work. Research which indicates, for example, that 'more training is needed' can be evaluated in relation to non-supportive environments, or outlines of feasible training programmes can be developed. A project looking at counselling skills, for example, would probably find that the research indicates that nurses are not skilled in this area, and that they need more training. The student could then relate this to his or her working environment; to the opportunities for training which exist there, and the other demands on the staff. Situations where increases in workload reduce educational time can be analysed in terms of the nature of the crisis, its origin, and the way it could be handled. In this way the crisis becomes an opportunity for developing knowledge about practice, and is a more productive way of coping with these problems. This type of work often leads the students away from the immediate situations of nurse-patient interaction, to organisational and political debates. This is not contrary to reflective practice, it is simply widening the scope of reflection to incorporate the wider context in which nursing takes place. The potential value of this is enormous, in that nurses may increase their understanding of these larger arenas in ways which can empower them.

Practice priorities cannot always be capitalised on in this way, but this does not mean that they are purely negative factors in nurse education. They constitute an essential part of nursing – the notion that patients matter. If patient care was not important, then nurse education would not be either. Practice priorities are part of the world which students work in, and as such they cannot be ignored or dismissed.

This is not to say that educational imperatives are irrelevant to practice, but they are certainly less pressing and less immediate than a crisis such as half of the ward staff being absent from work due to sickness. It has to be said, however, that even in situations where time out for staff education is possible, this is not always encouraged. Part of this problem probably arises from the suspicion that some nurses have about theory, a point discussed in the last chapter. This suspicion reduces the amount of support for students available in the clinical placement, and therefore, as with pre-registration students, makes the integration of theory and practice difficult to demonstrate by example. Mentorship schemes are an attempt to address this problem in Project 2000 courses, but a similar scheme is more difficult to establish for post-basic academic courses.

The reasons for this are several. Firstly there is a reluctance among staff to volunteer for this type of role, unless they have done such a course themselves. This reluctance appears to stem from a sense of inferiority, and a reluctance to expose themselves to potential embarrassment if their input is not sufficiently 'academic'.

There are also problems arising from the nature of the mentor-learner relationship. As the student is a permanent member of the staff a 'working relationship' exists, which is not necessarily seen by either party as appropriate for mentorship. If the relationship is based on equality of knowledge and power, then this balance can be disrupted by the student asking for help (seen as a subordinate position) or by the student's increase in knowledge (seen as conferring higher status). Even if the mentor is the student's manager, the balance of this relationship can be altered, or in some cases inequalities reinforced as the manager assumes control of the student's learning, and the student feels obliged to submit to this influence.

This role obviously needs a clearer definition. The usual portrayal of the mentor as someone from whom the student can learn from may need to change to emphasise the sharing and supportive aspects of the role. Developing this idea, however, is more problematic than in pre-registration courses, where there is a clearly defined pool of mentors within an established training circuit. Post-registration courses take students from many different units and Health Authorities, and typically these change from year to year. It is therefore difficult to hold workshops or meetings to discuss these issues, and it is unlikely that written information for students or mentors will address these complex points adequately.

This lack of exemplar mentors in the clinical environment places a greater burden on lecturers. They have to provide exemplars, support, and share experiences with the students. This does, however, create a problem for teachers, not only because they may feel uncomfortable with this ethos, but because they may feel that they do not fully belong to the world in which practice takes place, and consequently feel that they have little to say about it. The newly-developed post of lecturer/practitioner may go some way towards addressing this problem, however, as this role explicitly recognises the importance of continued practice. Until such appointments become the norm, teachers will still feel like 'visitors' in the clinical area. Being a 'visitor', however, can be an advantage, in that it can facilitate the acknowledgement of the more particular and specific knowledge students have of practice settings. This knowledge can be used as a resource for teaching, in such instances as presenting examples of practice problems, developing practicums, and creating a climate in which students can talk freely about the issues they face. In this sense teachers can learn from the students and, if they listen carefully, and with respect, can avoid their work becoming abstract and decontextualised.

CONCLUSION

The debates in this chapter indicate that developing reflective practice is a complex process. The central problem is the conflict between educational and clinical imperatives, a problem which cannot be easily resolved. Given this impasse, nurse teachers need to think creatively about how reflective practice can be developed, and how clinical imperatives can be handled. There is potential for these imperatives to be used imaginatively in nurse education, and indeed they should form the basis of any programme, for clinical imperatives are what nursing is all about.

Reflective practice would appear to be a productive approach to take in nurse education and practice, offering as it does a way to bridge the theory/practice gap. Support for the concept of reflective practice has been widespread in nursing, to the extent that it has almost become a cliché. Munby and Russell (1989) highlight this problem when they state that 'it is obvious that 'reflection' is on the brink of becoming ambiguous, if it has not already joined the ranks of educational catchwords' (p.76). The use of the term 'reflective practice' in nurse education demonstrates this ambiguity, in particular a degree of confusion between 'reflection-in-practice' (the process of framing and reframing while engaged in dealing with practice problems) and 'reflection-on-practice' (the retrospective analysis of practice that has been performed). Similarly, the phrase 'integrating theory and practice' is used synonymously with reflective practice, when what is advocated is actually similar to technical rationality – in other words the application of academically derived theory, largely unshaped and unadapted, to the complexities of practice.

Another misinterpretation is the use of the term reflection to describe self-disclosure by students of their innermost fears and anxieties. Whereas this may be desirable to a certain extent, the logic being that to know others you must first know yourself, this becomes problematic if these self disclosures become compulsory and assessed. The ethical problems presented by this strategy are legion.

These misinterpretations are understandable given some of the problems which are encountered when trying to implement Schon's findings. Schon's work does not, and was probably not intended to, provide clear cut guidelines for teaching. (This would be an example of technical rationality in itself!) Some basic principles, however, can be distilled from Schon's discussion, which are related to the role of the teacher and the nature of the learning environment.

If we look, for example, at the concept of the coach, we can see that this demands a different style of teaching than traditional approaches, one that is much more discursive and open. It also demands a degree of expertise in the teacher at dealing with practice problems, expertise that many teachers have lost in their years away from practice. This suggests two strategies. Firstly teachers should be allowed to identify and develop their chosen area of expertise, perhaps by having some practice commitment, but also by being allowed to stay teaching within their chosen area. This would mean that the common practice of moving tutors around to different areas of teaching would have to stop.

The second strategy would be to integrate practitioners much more into the educational system. This would not only involve establishing mentorship schemes, but also explicitly recognising the value of the practice-based knowledge that they have. Respecting this knowledge is less likely to produce anxiety in mentors, who will be so concerned with being 'caught out' while not following official theory, that they will be unable to transmit their 'theories-inaction'.

The practicum presents more problems for nurse education. As we have discussed, the clinical environment is not a practicum, and it is difficult to recreate this environment in an educational setting. Our strategy has been to compromise, to develop 'focused practicums', which deal only with limited aspects of practice. Examples of these are given in this book, in Sections Two and Three, and they have worked well in their own terms, but they cannot match the complexity of the real world. Having 'time out' to look at specific aspects of practice is, of course, valuable, but the integration of the understanding gained of one aspect, with other issues in practice must be explicitly rather than implicitly addressed.

Another strategy that we have used to overcome the problems of the clinical setting as a practicum is to develop strategies and mechanisms by which students can record incidents and issues in practice, and then discuss them later (see Section Four). This is not reflection-in-practice, but reflection-on-practice. This is possibly the most that any educational system can do, given that access to reflection-in-practice is constrained by the demands of hot action (Eraut 1985). What this strategy does do, however, is to develop in the students the habit of reflection, in other words they become accustomed to having their practice analysed by themselves and others. This strategy is dependent on the skills of teaching staff who, either in tutorials or group sessions, can act as exemplars to the students, drawing upon a variety of perspectives, and applying them to practice issues. The staff, therefore, can show the students how reflection can be practised.

Operationalising the concept of reflective practice, therefore, is not as simple as relying on the old technical rationality model, in that it demands a number of changes, in philosophy, organisation and content of teaching. We have found it to be very difficult, although extremely interesting, and are becoming increasingly uncomfortable with traditional approaches to teaching, although we recognise that they too have their value. Throughout the process of moving towards this style of teaching we have had a number of debates and discussions about teaching methods and styles, and we still don't agree completely about some things. But that is the nature of any change. We would rather that these disputes happen, and continue to happen, than we all followed unquestioningly ideas which we did not understand or support. Perhaps this is the essence of teaching reflective practice – that teachers constantly reflect on their practice too.

REFERENCES

Benner, P. (1984) *From Novice to Expert: Excellence and Power in Clinical Nursing*. Addison Wesley. California.

Eraut, M. (1985) Knowledge creation and knowledge use in professional contexts. *Studies in Higher Education*. **10 (2)**, 117–33

Fretwell, J.E. (1982) *Ward Teaching and Learning*. RCN, London.

Lawler, J. (1991) *Behind the Screens. Nursing, Somology, and the Problem of the Body*. Churchill Livingstone, Edinburgh.

Maslow, A. (1970) *Motivation and Personality*, 2nd edition. Harper and Row, New York.

Melia, K. (1987) *Learning and Working: The Occupational Socialization Of Nurses*. Tavistock, London.

Munby, H. and Russell, T. (1989) Educating the reflective teacher, an essay review of two books by Donald Schon. *Journal of Curriculum Studies*, **21 (1)**, 71-80.

Orem, D.E. (1980) *Nursing: Concepts of Practice*. 2nd edition. McGraw-Hill, New York.

Orton, H.D. (1981) *Learning Climate: A Study of the Role of the Ward Sister in Relation to Student Nurse Learning*. RCN, London.

Procter, S. (1989) The functioning of nursing routines in the management of a transient workforce. *Journal of Advanced Nursing*, **14**, 180-189.

Rogers, C. (1951) *Client-centred Therapy*. Houghton-Mifflin, Boston.

Roy, C. (1980) The Roy Adaptation model. In Riehl, J.P. and Roy, C. (eds) *Conceptual Models for Nursing Practice*. 2nd edition. Appleton Century Crofts, Norwalk, CT.

Schön, D.A. (1987) *Educating the Reflective Practitioner*. Jossey-Bass, California.

Section Two
Skills and Knowledge

Introduction

This section deals with strategies that we have developed to introduce basic skills and knowledge to students. This stage, we feel is the precursor to reflective practice. The topics that this section covers are Information Retrieval Skills, (Chapter Four) Statistics (Chapter Five), and Information Technology (Chapter Six). Many others could have been included, for example sociology, psychology, and the life sciences, which all require a basic understanding of their concepts, their focus, and their methodology, but we felt that the topics we have chosen provide perhaps the clearest examples of building up basic skills within our repertoire. They all involve an incremental model of learning, with advanced concepts being built onto basic knowledge as learning progresses. This progression, or order of learning, has been carefully thought through, and modified as we have found out more about the way that students learn.

Some of the initial learning is, by its nature, divorced from the world of practice. Introducing students to computers, for example, requires that they should be taught about disk operating systems, a concept which cannot draw upon clinical experience. Having said this, however, such knowledge is acquired through exercises and workbook, rather than by traditional lectures, and thus comes under the heading of experiential learning. As soon as possible, students are asked to complete exercises which are linked to the world of practice, for example using a patient information database, designed to reflect the information that a 'real' database would contain. In doing this they encounter problems and difficulties which they have to solve by drawing upon their basic knowledge.

The information retrieval package which we have developed, which is concerned with library and study skills, is slightly different. The learning environment is not an approximation of the clinical world, but an approximation of the academic world, in which the problems involve issues such as accessing and evaluating information. Students are therefore taken through a series of exercises to introduce them to the different ways of accessing material, and are then asked to do a literature search on a topic of interest to them, as if they were doing an essay. Although this package is in some ways divorced from practice, it also begins to introduce ideas about evaluating material and knowledge, a fundamental requisite for reflective practice. This represents a move from simply acquiring knowledge to learning how to use it. By encouraging students to examine literature more closely, the seeds of critical evaluation are sown.

4 An information retrieval and analysis package

David O'Brien and Graham Walton

INTRODUCTION

This chapter describes the development of an Information Retrieval Skills package (IRS). In many ways this package was crucial to the development of student-centred, androgogical approaches to nurse education within the nursing division at the University of Northumbria. It provided the foundation for the development of other student centred packages, especially the Clinical Studies assignment (Chapter 10) and the Interpersonal and Communication Skills package (Chapter 7).

The original package was completed in 1986 at which time it became part of the formal assessment strategy for the Diploma in Professional Studies in Nursing Course. It has subsequently been updated and modified on several occasions and is now a feature of all the pre- and post-registration nursing courses at the university. It has also been modified and adapted for several other courses both within the Department and outside the health studies area.

This chapter describes the development of this package and the contribution it makes to student-centred learning. It identifies the increasingly important role of the librarian as a resource person and facilitator of learning and highlights the need for lecturers to work with the librarian on the development, teaching and assessment of the package. The chapter concludes with a discussion of the strategies used to evaluate the package and of contemporary innovations in library-based information systems.

THE INFORMATION RETRIEVAL AND ANALYSIS PACKAGE

The package is usually given to students at the beginning of their course and therefore forms their first assignment.

With most courses there is a general introduction to the package given by both the lecturer and librarian together. This explores the purpose, schedule and weighting of the work. The librarian then has an hour-long session with groups of a maximum of fourteen students to introduce both the necessary skills and also the major relevant sources. There are time-tabled sessions in which students can work on the assignment. Emphasis is placed upon students being able to contact both the librarian and lecturer for individual help. The students usually submit the assignment towards the end of the first term. They are therefore given between 10 and 15 weeks to complete the assignment.

The information retrieval and analysis handbook has four sections:

1. Introduction to basic information retrieval skills;
2. Key concepts in nursing;
3. Professional development in nursing including nursing research and health education;
4. Official Government Reports.

The purpose of each section is set out below together with a sample of the activities included and a discussion of how each section contributes to the overall assessment.

Section One – An introduction to information retrieval skills

This section is concerned with a general orientation to the library and to fundamental skills of information retrieval.

The topics in this section include:

*   Geographical and physical location of library stock;
*   Key library staff;
*   Loan regulations;
*   Opening hours;
*   Reservations and inter-library loans;
*   Set text collection;
*   Photocopying and copyright law.

Systematic approaches to locating information in the library:

*   Microfiche catalogue;
*   Subject indexes;
*   Name – title indexes;
*   Classification systems;
*   Computer catalogue
*   Reference books;
*   Dictionaries;
*   Encyclopeadias;
*   Directories;
*   Year books;
*   In-house current awareness file;
*   Indexes and abstracts;
*   Bibliographic referencing;
*   Citation techniques;
*   Government publications.

The exercises completed in this section are formatively assessed and students are encouraged to work in small groups.

Section Two – Key concepts in nursing

This section is concerned with building upon the basic information retrieval and analysis skills and developing critical insight into the nature of a range of concepts fundamental to nursing theory and practice.

Examples of concepts addressed include pain, bereavement, sensory perception, communication, stress and anxiety. Two illustrative examples show how increasing conceptional development is expected within this section.

Example 1: Pain.

- Under which class numbers would you be able to locate information on the above topic?
- State the type of literature to be found under each class number.
- Using an appropriate bibliographic technique list three texts on the above topic.
- Using an appropriate bibliographical technique list three nursing research studies on the above topic.
- What do you understand by the term non-invasive methods of pain relief?
- List four different non-invasive methods of pain relief.

Example 2: Nurse-patient relationships.

- Under which class numbers would you be able to locate texts on the above topic?
- Using an appropriate bibliographical technique list ten texts on the above topic.
- Give a short account of any two nursing research studies on the above topic.
- Explain what is meant by the following:
  - non-verbal communication
  - verbal communication skills
  - attributes of a 'good' communicator
  - problems associated with nurse patient communication.

In each of the above all reference sources must be acknowledged.

Section Two is summatively assessed with a weighting of 25%.

Section Three – Professional development in nursing

This section includes a consideration of statutory framework for nursing, research in nursing and concepts of health. The skills developed in Section 2 are further developed within this section, for example it includes a consideration of concepts of health; here students are again expected to locate relevant information sources but in addition they are expected to appraise critically a research article or book chapter. The skills of criticism are addressed in study skills and research appreciation sessions on their course, and this package provides a useful way of reinforcing these skills.

Section Three is summatively assessed with a weighting of 35%.

Section Four – Government and official reports

In the final section students are expected to compare and contrast the conclusions of two major reports. Currently these are the Black report and the White Paper CMND 555 *Working for Patients*. This final assessment relies heavily upon students being able to use the critical skills developed in earlier sections. Issues such as ideology, freedom of speech and ethical neutrality are also addressed since these two reports are built upon vastly differing notions of health and the individual's and society's responsibilities. Again these concepts are covered in formal taught sessions, for example as part of social policy lectures, and the package helps to reinforce students' understanding of these ideas.

Section Four is summatively assessed and has a weighting of 40%.

THEORETICAL CONSIDERATIONS

The package is largely underpinned by behavioural and cognitive ideas of education. It is behaviourist in that information retrieval skills and analysis are broken down into discrete stages of learning which are structured so that understanding can develop progressively. There are two different strands to this progression. One is the progression in complexity of the sources used in information retrieval, from simple library catalogues, to the use of official publications. Understanding relatively straightforward concepts such as the Dewey Decimal system enables students to grasp the fundamental principles of organising material according to topic. They can then move on to looking at sources such as indexes and abstracts, which usually organise material according to topic, author, and date. From this stage they can then begin to access material from official publications which is organised under additional headings including source (i.e. Government department) and status (i.e. working party or Royal Commission).

The second way in which the workbook fosters progression is in the increasing complexity of the way in which students are asked to use material. They are initially asked simply to find material, they are then introduced to the principles of referencing (which clarifies the notion of plagiarism for the students), and then to describe or define material. From this descriptive stage they then move on to higher level skills such as summarising, classifying, comparing and contrasting material, and finally critically appraising it. The cognitive dimension is, therefore, introduced through the progression to critical analysis. Mastery of each stage is seen as a development towards this aim.

Behavioural learning theory has been very influential in nurse education. It is essentially reductionist as it assumes that complex learning activities can be broken down to simpler units and their completion measured directly (Alurip 1985). As such it has been criticised as being mechanistic and failing to capture the affective parts of learning. While valid, we would argue that this criticism does not render behavioural theory completely redundant. It may well be inappropriate to use this approach to inform learning in what might be called the affective domain (for example communication skills), however, we feel there is much to be said for organising some other types of learning in this way.

Information retrieval skills, we believe, is one such area. It is based on knowledge and understanding of library organisation, which can be developed incrementally from very basic to more complex skills. Mastering these stages through a clearly structured progressive assignment is a vital part of developing the student's ability to study. The importance of developing this skill is not, however, always recognised by students who frequently dismiss it as tedious, or unimportant. It is often only when they have difficulties in accessing information, later on in the course, that they realise that their lack of understanding will handicap them.

Introducing the IRS at the beginning of courses has helped to prevent students experiencing 'library madness', where the search for material becomes frantic, chaotic, and ultimately fruitless. Given that few students recognise the importance of mastering these skills the initial motivation to do this work lies in the fact it is summatively assessed, which means that it is a compulsory part of the course. This can be regarded as an extrinsic motivation but as the package also allows students to look at topics and issues they find interesting, this can provide some intrinsic motivation. Adopting a behavioural approach therefore recognises that some students will not have a burning desire to understand information retrieval skills, and so provides a means of encouraging students to tackle this area of knowledge.

Combining information retrieval skills with analysis is not without its problems. Essentially the information retrieval element of the package needs to be mastered as early as possible in the course so that the skills learnt can be utilised in subsequent assignments. It is difficult, however, to master critical analysis in the first term of a diploma course. Indeed we would see mastery of this skill as the ultimate goal of the whole course. Like all of the early assignments in courses which utilise continuous assessment, the IRS is both formative and summative. It is formative in that it provides a structured approach to mastering essential skills and summative in that it is assessed. While we recognise that few of the students will master critical analysis within this assignment, it provides a structured approach to some of the basic skills of analysis, such as summarising, categorising and contrasting material. These skills are transferable to all other assignments on the course and we feel that practising these skills early on in the course enhances the students' subsequent work. It also provides an opportunity for feedback to the student on these basic skills.

Within continuous assessment it is possible to argue that all early assignments which aim to develop analytical skills should be formative, as the students have not yet mastered these skills. However, without a summative assessment some will never try. The students' lack of ability in the area of critical analysis during initial assignments can perhaps best be tackled through the weighting given to the assignment when determining the final award.

PRACTICAL CONSIDERATIONS

Over the years the IRS package has given rise to a variety of issues. Perhaps the most important issue is that of resources. These are not only financial, but human too. The package is supported by librarians and academic staff who need to be familiar with the expectations of students' performances. It also requires supporting lectures, seminars and tutorials and can, therefore, be very labour intensive. In addition it is highly dependent upon good team work and communication between lecturers and librarians. These human resources, however, are insufficient if library sources are inadequate. If the library cannot offer a range of learning experiences in terms of retrieval systems, or if it does not have a large enough range and quantity of material, then any learning package designed will be correspondingly limited.

Shared learning

Other issues concern the student's approach to learning. As it is the first assignment that is assessed on the course some students regard it as an examination. In other words they view it as a test of ability which must be completed unaided – any assistance is regarded as 'cheating'. These students have difficulty, therefore, in reconciling the fact that the staff who assess the assignment can also give them significant help in completing it. They are therefore reluctant to seek advice as they assume that either the staff will not give it, or such a request will be regarded as a indicator of low ability. The lecturer is regarded with suspicion by some students, as someone who will be ever vigilant in the detection of incompetence, and as a person to whom no weakness must be admitted.

These ideas can be explained through people being unfamiliar with androgogical concepts. Knowles (1978) has outlined how, in adult education, the teacher becomes more involved with enabling rather then directing the student. This, however, can be a difficult idea for some students and some staff to grasp. These concerns are not, however, specific to this package but reflect issues which arise generally in relation to student-centred learning and continuous assessment. From this perspective, therefore the assignment also provides a useful introduction to supervision.

Similarly some students can also be uncomfortable with the idea of collaborating with their peers. This is generally encouraged, echoing Knowles' (1978) emphasis on the usefulness of the student group in the learning process. Students, however, can be very territorial about their work, and are often reluctant to share it, some seeing this as a form of cheating or laziness. It must be admitted that this also creates a dilemma for staff assessing the work. If this 'sharing' occurs with all sections of the workbooks its value as a learning exercise will be diminished. Various methods have been used to resolve this issue. Information skills concerned with summarising, comparison and analysis are given a heavier weighting than those of, say, finding a definition in a dictionary. Thus it becomes subject to the same principles of assessment which cover essay writing and it would be hoped that any plagarism either from texts or from another student would be picked up by the normal processes of internal and external examining. Another approach is to make those sections in which the same answer is required from every student into a formative assessment with only the remainder being summative.

Student-centred learning – a balanced approach

As discussed earlier the package is designed to develop the students skills of critical analysis. For many students this is difficult and a balance has to be struck between promoting independent learning and providing feedback while the student is completing the assignment in order to facilitate this skill. In fact a case can be made for formatively assessing each section of the workbook before allowing the student to proceed to the next section. This ensures that any problems are picked up early and not repeated throughout the entire assignment. It must also be recognised that the skills of critical analysis are difficult to learn and tend to generate considerable anxiety among students. When linked to a package such as this students can become so immersed in the minutiae of the assignment that they forget its purpose. Some students become so anxious that they cannot differentiate between significant skills and those that are less important. In these circumstances issues like the difference between a 'reference list' and a 'bibliography' can take on gargantuan proportions. Staff have to be aware of this and provide a sense of proportion.

A balance has to be achieved, therefore, between allowing students to learn through the experience of the assignment and ensuring they are given sufficient initial guidance to start them off. The worst possible scenario would be for a student to be alienated from libraries as a direct result of having to complete the assignment without adequate initial or continuing preparation.

The role of the librarian

Teaching information skills in this manner has a major impact upon the librarian's work. Not only is it time consuming to plan the work, teach the skills and mark the work but there is also a commitment to evaluate the experience and attend the relevant course committees. Provision of extra library staff to support these activities is unlikely so the librarian must cope with this on top of everything else.

If this learning is to be successful it needs to be a joint venture between the librarian and the lecturer. The librarian must ensure that it is not taken over by academic staff. In order for librarians to be able to do this they need to have subject expertise, an understanding of educational processes, be proactive and have a tactful manner as well as what are perceived as 'traditional' librarian skills. Librarians are placed in the unenviable position of being needed to help answer queries in the library, assess students' work, attend course planning committees and course committees and also teach in the classroom.

Apart from the time taken with marking completed work there is another implication. Students who have spent a lot of time and effort in their information skills work and have not achieved a reasonable mark i.e. not been 'rewarded' for their effort, can feel aggrieved and will need an explanation. Having to counsel students in this area is a new experience for many librarians. It does, however, high-light that they need to be able to justify their marking and be prepared to give lengthy personal feedback to individual students if it is requested.

THE PROCESS OF EVALUATION

In an ideal world, when a library instruction programme is planned, careful consideration will take place about how its effectiveness can be evaluated and monitored. The fundamental purpose of evaluation as identified by Astin and Panos (1971) is to collect/analyse information that can be used for rational educational decision making. In a seminal article, Werking (1980) argues that evaluation is important to assess both the overall effectiveness and also the methods of instruction. There are three groups for whom feedback about the programme is essential: the library staff, academic staff and the students. Fjallbrant and Malley (1983) state that evaluation should be multi-faceted and involved with 'library use and information skills, attitudes to libraries, effects of various instructional programmes, and use of given library or information resources'.

This is all very laudable but in reality evaluation is very often ignored when information skills programmes are established. There are a variety of reasons for this. Hanson (1984) has identified a number of factors. Firstly the limited class contact between librarians and students means that the librarian does not get to know the students sufficiently to establish the level of their prior experience, particularly as the IRS is usually undertaken at the beginning of the course. Secondly producing/analysing tests and questionnaires is very time-consuming and needs careful thought. Thirdly, the students may not initially appreciate the importance of information retrieval skills to their overall ability to complete the course. Therefore, the type of evaluation used – and the timing of the evaluation – may have heavy and, in some cases, quite negative influence on the outcome. These factors indicate that evaluation can be an arduous and potentially disheartening experience. It is not surprising, then, that in many cases there is a reliance solely on informal feedback gained from students and staff.

Evaluation takes on increased importance when the students' information skills are being formally assessed and the library becomes more central to the learning process. Under these circumstances it is important that factors which affect the learning process in a negative way are identified. While not claiming to be paragons of virtue, we have tried a wide range of methods and this variety indicates that the ideal method has not yet been found.

Approaches to evaluation

Two major approaches to evaluation can be identified – an experimental approach and a more qualitative approach. With the experimental approach two or more identical groups of students are established. The information skills level of all the students is identified initially through some form of test. One group completes a library instruction programme and a post test is then administered to both groups and any resulting difference is identified. We have used this approach in our evaluations, for example Greenfield (1987) adapted the workbook for use at Sunderland School of Nursing (now Bede College) and conducted an experimental evaluation. Three separate groups of students were compared, with the workbook being given to two of the groups. All three then undertook exercises using the School of Nursing library. It was found that the two groups who had completed the workbook answered the questions more accurately and quickly than the third group. This method can be criticised for considering outcomes only. It gives no information on the strengths and weaknesses of the workbook as it is currently constructed. It is, therefore, much more product-orientated rather than process-orientated.

For these reasons subsequent approaches at the University of Northumbria have been more qualitative. This recognises that most health courses at the university are based on the process curriculum model. As Kelly (1982) has pointed out it is important that the evaluation techniques used must be congruent with the curriculum model. Confusion will result if evaluation techniques based on the product model are applied to the process curriculum. It follows, therefore, that as the curriculum and information skills workbook is based on experiential and discovery methods, sympathetic evaluation techniques had to be developed.

One approach we have adopted is to develop an open-ended questionnaire in which students are asked to evaluate their own level of confidence with ten specific information skills. This enables areas which require further attention to be identified. Typically students are happy about finding classification numbers, locating journal articles and writing a reference but are not so sure about citation techniques and government publications (O'Brien et al. 1990; Procter 1988; Walton 1989).

Similarly a questionnaire is used to evaluate the information skills workbook completed by the BSc. Occupational Therapy students (Lyne and Walton 1990). Again this establishes the students' level of confidence in information retrieval skills. It also investigates the perceived support given to students, and identifies where else in the course the skills have been applied as well as the changes the students would like to make to the assignment.

The method which has produced some of the richest data is the nominal group technique. This technique was devised by Delbecq (1975) and allows a group's views to be established without input from the evaluator. It avoids pre-conceptions about what the students may or not consider important and also stops a single individual's views from dominating the group. This method was used at the beginning and after six months of the course to look at students' views on information sources (Walton 1989). Students started with a preconception that lecturers would be the most important source but after six months other sources had a higher profile, which indicates a pleasing increase in student independence.

It is fair to point out that some information skills are still only evaluated on an informal basis. Decisions are reached about changes over coffee or through passing comments in the Library. Hanson (1984) found that if the evaluation of the information skills is not written into the course there is no automatic means of obtaining feedback. The only guaranteed way to ensure evaluation occurs is to consider it at the core of the programme. Sessions to complete the evaluation need to be built into the timetable. The techniques should be piloted and planned so they can function smoothly. Once the findings have been produced all parties, including students as well as lecturers and librarians, need to be allowed to assess their significance and discuss resulting changes.

The introduction of a structured and planned process of evaluation reduces the temptation to completely re-design the workbook on the basis of idiosyncratic results obtained from one group of students. At the university all evaluations are considered together and updates undertaken only when those staff who are primarily responsible for the workbook feel that sufficient progress has been made in refining the ideas behind it to warrant substantive changes.

FUTURE DEVELOPMENTS

The potential for expansion of the teaching of information skills is enormous. At the present time two major innovations are being assessed; one is concerned with using a modified information skills package as part of an entry gate into advanced nurse education courses and the other centres upon a computer system known as CD-ROM.

Entry gate into advanced nurse education

It is a misnomer that information skills are low-order skills in nursing. For example they can range from using the index of a book to down loading CD-ROM search and manipulating the references with database and word processing software. By identifying the level of the course it is possible to structure an information skills programme to the appropriate standard. This flexibility means it can be adapted for a number of circumstances. When selecting students for post-registration courses there is sometimes a need for students to improve their skill level in certain areas before they start the course. Initial plans have started to produce an information skills workbook that address basic skills for certain prospective students to ensure that when they start the course they have achieved a minimum standard.

CD-ROM

The teaching of information skills takes on a new dimension with the introduction of the compact disk read only memory (CD-ROM). At present CD-ROM disks will hold about 550 million characters or the equivalent of 275,000 pages. The major nursing database *Cumulative Index to Nursing and Allied Health Literature* (CINAHL) is available in this format as well as the large medical database *Medline*. The CD-ROM has various advantages over the printed version which include records having abstracts, speed in searching and flexibility in search techniques. The problems posed in training users to a satisfactory level deserve a chapter to themselves.

Whitsed (1989) has identified the objectives of CD-Rom training sessions:

- To understand the reasons for choosing between the manual, online and CD-ROM version for a particular search;
- To understand the difference between natural language and controlled thesaurus searching.
- To introduce the functions of searching, printing, storing searches, downloading and exchanging discs.
- To understand the basic keyboard skills, including the use of function keys, enter key and cursor control arrows.

This list outlines the complex skills needed to be an efficient searcher. Formal training sessions are arranged for specific courses at the University of Northumbria as well as informal one to one demonstrations as requested. Neither of these methods is an ideal way to cover the areas. Following the success of the information retrieval skills package we have developed a workbook specifically on CD-ROM. The development of data sources such as the CD-ROM highlights the importance of students being able to match their information needs with the appropriate information source.

CONCLUSION

The IRS package has had a substantial impact on teaching and learning styles both within the Institute of Health Studies at the university and in Bede College. In both institutions it now forms the introductory assignment on most of the courses. As a consequence the students quickly learn how to use the library and are able to access a whole range of information on a variety of topics. This skill is utilised throughout the rest of the course. As lecturers we have found that on completion of the package most of the students tend to be less dependent on set books and more independent in their ablity to utilise available literature.

Major changes in the structure, organisation and orientation of nurse education discussed in Chapter One has resulted in the need to prepare students for a commitment to life long professional learning. The ability to access and critically appraise information sources is crucial to this process. The introduction of this package, early on in the students' education, provides a sound foundation for developing these abilities and graphically illustrates to students the vast range of material available to them on virtually any topic.

REFERENCES

Alurip, R. (1985) Learning theories and bibliographic instructions. In Kirkendall, C.A. (ed.) *Bibliographic Instruction and the Learning Process*. Piorian Press, Ann Arbor: 15–27.

Astin, A.W. and Panos, R.J. (1971) The evaluation of educational programs. In Thorndike, R.L. (ed.) *Education Measurement* 2nd ed. pp.733–751. American Council of Education, Washington.

Black D (1980). *Working Group on inequalities in Health*. Department of Health and Social Security, London.

Command S.S.S. (1989) *Working for Patients*. HMSO, London.

Delbecq, A. (1975) *Group Techniques for Programme Planning*. Scott F. Foreman & Co., Glenview.

Fjallbrant, N. and Malley, I. (1983) Evaluation in a user education programme. *User Education in Libraries* 2nd ed., pp.94–111. Clive Bingley, London.

Greenfield, M. (1987) The rationale, development and evaluation of an information retrieval skills package as a teaching strategy. Unpublished Project; Bede College of Nursing and Midwifery, Sunderland.

Hanson, J.R. (1984) Evaluation of library user education with reference to the programme at Dorset Institute of Higher Education. *Journal of Librarianship*, **16**, 1–18.

Kelly, A.V. (1982) *The Curriculum: Theory and Practice*. Harper and Row, London.

Knowles, M. (1978) *The Adult Learner*. Gulf Publishing, Houston.

Lyne, S. and Walton, G. (1990) Integrating information skills into a Diploma in Occupational Therapy Course. *British Journal of Occupational Therapy*, **53**, 92–4.

O'Brien, D. Procter, S. and Walton, G. (1990) Towards a strategy for teaching information skills to student nurses. *Nurse Education Today*, **10**, 125–9.

Procter, S. (1988) An evaluation of an information skills for nurses package. Unpublished Project; Institute of Health Sciences, University of Northumbria.

Walton, G. (1989) Effectiveness of library user education methods in health sciences courses at Newcastle upon Tyne Polytechnic. Unpublished thesis as part of MA Education Development Course; Department of Education, Newcastle upon Tyne Polytechnic.

Werking, R.H. (1980) Evaluating bibliographic education; a review and critique. *Library Trends*, **29**, 153–172.

Whitsed, N. (1989) CD-ROM an end user training tool? The experience of using Medline in a small medical school. *Library Program*, **23**, 117–126.

5 A statistics package

Bob Heyman and Steven Campbell

INTRODUCTION

The learning package discussed in this chapter is the second in a series of four statistical packages, developed in the Institute of Health Sciences at the University of Northumbria, which take students from an elementary level to advanced multivariate statistics. This chapter provides an overview of the package and discussion of the resources required, both in terms of staff and equipment, to use the package for teaching purposes. It is important to note at the outset that this chapter is only really relevant for those who already teach statistics and therefore possess a good understanding of statistical techniques. The package discussed in this chapter is not designed for the novice teacher. It is aimed at the experienced teacher of statistics who is looking for new and creative ways to teach a subject that has traditionally tended to confound most nursing students.

An overview of the four packages

This section briefly outlines the content of each of the four packages. The approximate hours of classroom teaching required by each package is indicated in brackets. The first package (8 hours) involves students in using calculators to work out simple formulae and descriptive statistics, such as means and standard deviations. The second package (16 hours), to be discussed in detail in this chapter, introduces the use of inferential statistics to analyse relationships between two variables, using the statistical computer program, MINITAB. The third package (20 hours) uses MINITAB to analyse relationships between variables using real survey data, derived from the Health and Lifestyle Survey (Blaxter 1990). It extends the students' repertoire of statistical techniques, teaches them how to choose the most appropriate test and increases their awareness of problems and pitfalls in interpreting statistical results. The fourth package (20 hours) uses another statistical program, SPSS-PC, to introduce techniques of multivariate analysis.

Taken together, the packages provide students with progressively more advanced levels of understanding of statistics. Students on the Diploma of Nursing, for example, take the first two packages in order to enhance their critical understanding of published research. Postgraduate students at MSc or PhD level would be expected to take all four packages as part of their research training.

The focus in the packages is upon 'classical' inferential statistics rather than, for example, exploratory data analysis or Bayesian statistics. The reason for this is that the vast majority of published quantitative nursing research presently uses classical techniques. As the course aims to assist students both in critically evaluating published research as well as contributing to its development, it seemed sensible to concentrate on classical techniques at least in the initial packages. These packages will be modified to reflect future developments in nursing research as these arise.

'Classical' inferential statistics assumes a random sample. In practice this is rarely achieved in social research, including research into nursing. The classical techniques are still important, however, because they can indicate what conclusions could be drawn if the sample was approximately random. These conclusions can be distinguished from those about the randomness of the sample.

Material on statistical inference should be linked to discussion of the practicalities of sampling, problems in obtaining random samples in real research and the limitations that non-random samples impose upon interpretation. A middle way has to be found between an idealised text book account which ignores the barriers to achieving random samples and a purist approach which rejects inference from any sample which is less than perfectly random. Social research, including nursing research, is the art of interpreting imperfect data.

WHY THE LEARNING PACKAGE WAS NEEDED

Our discussion here will focus on the second learning package. This introduces techniques of statistical inference for two variables, using chi squared and 't' tests as examples. The third package demonstrates that similar principles can be applied to other tests of relationship between two variables (e.g. correlation, Mann-Whitney test).

Both of the authors failed to comprehend statistics courses during their under-graduate studies and found that the 'light dawned' only when forced to apply statistical techniques to data they collected while undertaking their own research. Experience over many years with students who have taken conventional courses in statistics has convinced us that we are a representative sample in this respect!

Several reasons can be identified for the comprehension problem, including anxiety about mathematics, the complexity of the logic underlying statistical inference and the gap between classroom examples of statistical problems and their application in real research. Nurses entering higher education, whether at Diploma, Degree or Postgraduate level, have problems which are no different to those of other students, e.g. undergraduate sociologists. However, part-time and mature students are more likely to suffer anxiety blocks.

Educational rationale

Use of a statistical computer program for teaching purposes has a number of advantages:

1. It allows probability theory to be tested empirically through students selecting random samples from a known population;
2. It frees students from having to struggle with calculation at the same time as they try to grasp statistical principles;
3. It introduces students to the practicalities of the use of computers in statistical analysis.

The first point requires further discussion. Classical inferential statistics involves comparing the observed relationship in an actual sample with the relationships which would be likely to occur if the variables were unrelated in the population. Our experience has shown that most students find this concept difficult to grasp and that it is easy for statistics teachers to underestimate the difficulty. However, once they have grasped the principle they can readily apply it to other statistical tests of the relationship between two variables.

The foundation of the learning package is a series of exercises which require students to select many random samples from a population with known parameters and to plot chance distributions as a class. The course starts with the simple and familiar example of estimating the voting intentions of a population on the basis of random samples. Data about the voting behaviour of every resident of a fictitious ward are entered onto the computer, by the lecturer, prior to the start of course. The database consists of 4000 residents half of whom vote Conservative and half Labour. Each student draws a series of random samples consisting of 100 residents from the parent population during the taught sessions. These samples are all taken at the same time by the students. The students are made aware of the content of the database and therefore the difference between their random samples and the parent population from which it is drawn, is graphically illustrated. This exercise is used to illustrate the principles of random sampling.

The data collected by all of the students is then pooled. This demonstrates the principles of distribution and the tendency for population samples to cluster around the mean. The Appendix to this chapter is an extract from the workbook detailing this aspect of the course.

Only after a thorough empirical demonstration of probability principles, involving the pooling of data and classroom discussion, are students expected to consider real statistical problems involving samples and unknown population parameters. The real problems need to engage the interest of the group and are drawn therefore from real health research e.g. the relationship between lead absorption in children and their behaviour.

TEACHING REQUIREMENTS

Teaching requires a laboratory with one terminal per student. The set up could be, for example, a network of peripheral terminals connected to a main-frame or central computer, a local area network, or even stand alone computers. As will be discussed below, individual practice outside formal teaching is essential. This requires both that a laboratory is available for casual use and that students have space in their timetable to work individually.

Ideally, it should be possible for students to echo their keyboard input to the printer in order to produce a printout of their work during the session which can be studied later. The command for this in MINITAB is 'outfile "output" '(see the Appendix to this chapter). However, we have also found it useful to include a correct version of the output in the workbooks. This can be compared with the screen or printed output. Students are reassured when they find that they have correctly carried out the commands and achieved the result identified in the workbook. The workbook copy of the output can also be used by students who get into difficulties during the session and are therefore unable to complete an exercise, or who are unable to attend a session.

Software requirements include an interactive statistical program (e.g. MINITAB, SPSS-PC, SYSTAT or SAS) and the data and macro files to be used in the workbook. It is crucial that the program is interactive. Batch programs, such as SPSS-X, are unsuitable for initial learning because of the complexity of their operation. Some issues about the choice of program will be discussed in the section on future developments (see page 64).

The number of students needs to be matched to the number of terminals in the laboratory and large groups will need to be split up for teaching purposes. Students spend much of their time interacting individually with the statistical program. A low staff/student ratio is required, particularly at the beginning of the course, in order to provide reasonably prompt responses to individual problems. We have found that a ratio of 12 students to one tutor is needed even after students have had time to get used to working with the computer. In the first stage of the course, extra assistance is helpful.

Because the course is based on a workbook it is relatively easy for teaching staff to familiarise themselves with the exercises and act as assistants even if their own grasp of statistics is limited. Several of our assistants have reported that helping with this exercise has been a learning experience for them and that they have finally realised what statistics is about! However, it is essential that both the course leader and the assistants practise and test the exercises thoroughly in advance of the class.

TEACHING METHODS

Teaching is organised around the workbook (see end of chapter for extracts). The workbook includes the following:

1. Theoretical material which can be read by students before the session and used as the basis for classroom discussion.
2. Instructions for the use of the statistical program. Explicit 'cookbook' instructions are provided when commands are first introduced. Subsequent exercises require students to adapt commands which have been

introduced and so require active learning.
3. Individual exercises which require students to write solutions into the workbook.
4. Class exercises which require students to pool data, for example on the results of sampling.

The workbook is used to structure each of the taught sessions and to determine the content. Formal lecturing is kept to a minimum and is undertaken as far as possible at the start of each session. It is concerned mainly with a review of the progress made to date and the introduction of new material. Deliberate repetition in class of material worked on in the previous session is used to consolidate and reinforce learning. An informal question and answer method encourages students to think actively about what they have learnt and reveals gaps in their understanding.

Students spend most of their time working individually. The material to be covered during the session will be identified from the workbook at the beginning of each session. It is important that the pace of sessions is set to that of the slowest students and it is easy for lecturers to overestimate how much can be achieved in a given time. The quicker students are encouraged to help the slower ones when they have completed their own work. They usually enjoy doing this but can be somewhat intolerant of their colleagues' mistakes!

We have found that two hours is the optimum length of time for a teaching session. This allows time for about half an hour of initial discussion and 90 minutes of practical work. The pace should be reasonably slow. Students should be encouraged to adopt a relaxed attitude, to take short breaks and to finish early if they experience fatigue.

Students should be advised to practise outside the formal class. By working in small groups, they can pool their knowledge and skills and learn to solve problems without relying on teaching staff. It should be possible, however, to summon a lecturer if the group is unable to solve a problem. In our experience, doing exercises without the physical presence of a lecturer increases the students' confidence, stimulates active learning and is the key to mastery of statistical principles. Students will often report that they 'wasted' time through being unable to get a command to work. They should be advised that this is an inevitable part of learning to use a computer individually and that they will eventually become fluent users of the system.

The material in the workbook is cumulative. Major problems occur if individuals miss sessions. Students need to be encouraged to attend every session and to catch up individually if they are unable to attend, enlisting the help of other students or tutors if necessary.

EVALUATION

Evaluation has included student questionnaires and feedback at course reviews. The most recent feedback has been very positive, but there were problems with early versions of the packages. One problem is that students are required to master computer skills and statistical skills simultaneously.

This can lead to 'cognitive overload' unless the presentation of material is handled with care. As indicated above, we have found it useful to have review sessions at the start of each class in order to look back at what was learnt in the last session as well as to introduce new material.

Some problems have arisen from developments in hardware and software. For example, one group had to move from an antiquated Harris computer to a Vax computer when the former was taken out of service. The change over could not be avoided but was not appreciated by students.

Hardware capacity has been another problem leading to excessively long response times from the computer network. The use of mini computer and main frame based software has meant that students have not been able to transfer these skills to their own workplace.

When the packages were initially developed in the mid 1980s, the only computer based means of statistical processing available to us were through MINITAB on a mini or mainframe computer and SPSS-X on a mainframe computer. MINITAB on a mini computer was used for all of the learning packages except the advanced course in multivariate analysis. SPSS-X had to be used for the advanced course as multivariate techniques are not available in MINITAB. There was considerable student complaint about having to switch both hardware and software. We are now able to offer advanced courses on IBM compatible micro-computers using SPSS-PC. This is a much more friendly environment and skills acquired can be transferred more easily to other settings.

FUTURE DEVELOPMENTS

The learning packages are still under active development. We intend both to modify existing packages and to produce new ones.

One development will be to use SPSS-PC for all the learning packages. MINITAB cannot be used for the advanced work on multivariate analysis. There is a dilemma between giving students the opportunity to sample more than one statistical program and facilitating learning by using one program only. Given the difficulty which many students experience, we favour using one program throughout.

A minor but important change will be to break up the manuals more clearly into individual lessons, so that the target for each session is clear. This can only be done on the basis of experience of how much the slowest students can realistically achieve in one session.

New packages will focus on the use of computer programs for the representation of descriptive statistics. Experience with more advanced research students has shown that they tend to neglect descriptive statistics in favour of inferential statistics, because they imagine that the latter are more 'scientific'. The techniques to be covered include graphical representation, tables and epidemiological measures, such as odds and standardised ratios. Students will be taught how to interface statistical programs with spreadsheets, presentation graphics programs and wordprocessors.

CONCLUSION

This book is aimed at nurses and those who teach them. The learning packages discussed in this chapter were developed for health professionals in general and can be used for a wide variety of groups who are interested in social behaviour. The only real adaptation necessary is in the choice of examples as these must be seen by students as relevant and interesting.

The use of learning packages based on statistical programs has advantages and disadvantages as with any other educational strategy. This particular strategy places great demands on the students in terms of both comprehension and skill. The difficulty involved in initially grasping statistical principles cannot be underestimated. By contrast, it is relatively easy to apply these principles to new statistical tests. The techniques that we have outlined are aimed at generating a deeper understanding of the principles of statistics. The sessions require considerable preparation by the lecturers concerned both in the form of workbooks and the installation of data bases and statistical packages onto the computer which are accessed by the students during the taught sessions. We feel that the greater level of understanding achieved by the students more than compensates for any increased workload that this method of teaching imposes on teachers, and in some cases, students.

REFERENCES

Blaxter, M. (1990) *Health and Lifestyles*, Routledge, London.

Appendix to Chapter 5

EXTRACTS FROM MANUAL INTRODUCTION TO INFERENTIAL STATISTICS USING MINITAB

We will now go into MINITAB (a program which performs statistical analysis) by:

MINITAB
OUTFILE 'OUTPUT'

The OUTFILE command is used to make a copy of the output which can be printed, as will be explained at the end of the session. When you go into MINITAB you should always set an outfile.

AN EXERCISE IN SAMPLING

For this exercise we will consider a simplified ward (Simpleton) which has 4000 voters, 50% of whom vote Conservative (1) and 50% of whom vote Labour (2). We will generate the 'data' for the population by:

SET C1
2000(1,2)

We can obtain a frequency distribution for the entire population with the following commands (including the punctuation exactly as shown):

TALLY C1;
ALL.

As you can see, Simpleton is a very marginal constituency! Let us suppose that a researcher does not have access to the population data and wishes to estimate the voting intentions of a random sample of Simpleton voters. A numerical description of a population is referred to as a PARAMETER. An estimate of the population parameter based on a sample is referred to as a STATISTIC. By convention, parameters are given Greek symbols and statistics are given Roman symbols. In this case:

POPULATION PROPORTION=π=50%=.5
SAMPLE PROPORTION
SIZE OF SAMPLE (NUMBER OF CASES)=N

Usually, like the opinion pollster who cannot afford to poll all the voters in a constituency, we would not know the population parameter. If we did, statistical inference would be unnecessary. With a real research problem we would only have a single small random sample from which to estimate the population parameter. For this exercise which is intended to illustrate principles of sampling, we will consider a population where P is known and we take many random samples.

We will use MINITAB to select a random sample of size 100 and compare the true population proportion with the sample estimate by:

SAMPLE 100 FROM C1 PUT INTO C2
TALLY C2;
ALL.

By subtracting the proportion of Conservative voters from 50, ignoring the sign, you can see the amount of error in your sample estimate. Each sample will probably give a different answer depending on which cases you happened to pick. Although its easy to work out the difference between π and P in this simple example, we will get MINITAB to do it for us as we will be generating a large number of samples in the next exercise.

We can do this by:

COPY C2 C3;
USE C2=1.
LET K1=ABSOLUTE(COUNT(C3)-50)
PRINT K1

This will affect C3 as illustrated below:

C2	C3
1	1
1	1
2	1
2	1

etc. etc.

Note: The SAMPLE command involves sampling without replacement. Providing that the sample N is low in comparison with the population N as would be the case in most social research we do not need to worry about this. Otherwise we would have to apply a 'finite population correction factor'.

So far we have just considered one sample as would be the case with a real piece of research where we did not know P. To see what typically happens when we take a sample we need to consider many samples. In order to avoid having to type in the commands again and again to produce samples we will use a 'macro' file. This is simply a stored set of commands which can be executed as if from the keyboard.

Produce 20 estimates of the sample deviation from 50%, writing each down as it is produced, by:

EXEC 'SAMMAC1' 20

As the answers come onto the screen, tally them in the SAMMAC1 column on the data sheet below. After you have recorded whatever is on the screen, respond **Y** to the CONTINUE? prompt in order to produce some more output.

DATA SHEET FOR CHANCE DIFFERENCES IN SAMPLE PROPORTIONS		
RANGE	FREQUENCY SAMMAC1	FREQUENCY SAMMAC2
0 – 0.9999	——	——
1 – 1.9999	——	——
2 – 2.9999	——	——
3 – 3.9999	——	——
4 – 4.9999	——	——
5 – 5.9999	——	——
6 – 6.9999	——	——
7 – 7.9999	——	——
8 – 8.9999	——	——
9 – 9.9999	——	——
10 – 10.9999	——	——
11 – 11.9999	——	——
12 – 12.9999	——	——
13 – 13.9999	——	——
14 – 14.9999	——	——
15 +	——	——

We can now enter the results for the entire class into the histogram below.

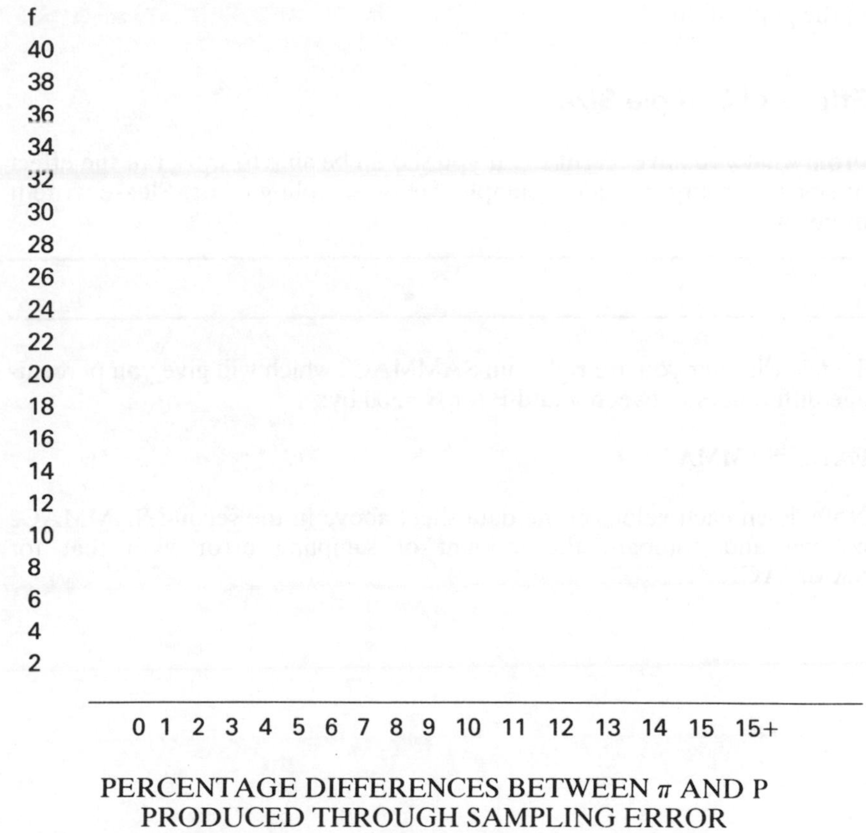

f
40
38
36
34
32
30
28
26
24
22
20
18
16
14
12
10
8
6
4
2

0　1　2　3　4　5　6　7　8　9　10　11　12　13　14　15　15+

PERCENTAGE DIFFERENCES BETWEEN π AND P
PRODUCED THROUGH SAMPLING ERROR

Fig. 5.1 Frequency distribution of chance differences between π and P

By smoothing the graph we can see that it has certain properties which are important for statistical inference:
  a.　Most sample estimates are quite close to π;
  b.　Large differences between π and P are unlikely;
  c.　The smoothed distribution has a known regular shape (called the binomial distribution).

The key idea behind statistical inference can be derived from this distribution. In real life social research we only have one sample and do not know the population parameter. However, we can estimate mathematically the point at which chance differences between the statistic and the parameter tail off and become unlikely. For example, if the difference between the Conservatives and Labour in the sample was 3% it would be quite probable that the true difference between them in the population could be 0. On the other hand, a difference of 10% occurs only rarely by chance. If the Conservatives were 10% ahead of Labour in the sample we could be almost certain that they were ahead in the population.

Effects of Sample Size

From what you have learnt so far you should be able to work out the effect of smaller or larger random sample size on sampling error. Please write it in below:

_____

_____

To test whether you are right run SAMMAC2 which will give you percentage differences between π and P for N=500 by:

EXEC 'SAMMAC2' 10

Note down each value on the data sheet above in the second SAMMAC2 column and compare the amount of sampling error with that for SAMMAC1.

6 An information technology package

Joan Aarvold, Bob Heyman, Brian Bell

INTRODUCTION

Information technology (IT) is becoming increasingly important in health care services. The information collected about patients is becoming more complex and is used for many different purposes. Nurses, as part of this computerised Health Service, will need to become proficient in the use of the new technologies. It appears however, that IT is a neglected part of the curriculum in pre- and post-registration courses. Part of this problem may be that such teaching requires levels of expertise and equipment which have not been part of the resources of centres for nurse education (Chambers and Coates 1990). There are also difficulties when embarking on a training programme in finding funding or choosing wisely from the range of computer hard and software available.

Nursing is therefore trapped – it cannot develop this expertise because it does not have this expertise. The consequences of neglecting IT, however, are potentially disastrous for the profession. Not only will nurses be unable to participate actively in the communication system of their organisation, but they will also find themselves unable to participate in the decisions made about the systems. How and what information is collected, and how it should be used are key issues for nurses as they plan for and make claims on resources. There is a danger that having spent years trying to escape the role of the doctor's handmaiden, nurses may now find themselves becoming the programmer's handmaiden.

The importance of IT training for all health care professionals is reinforced by government directives which provide frameworks for information systems and proposes strategies for training (Post White Paper, DoH Reports of Project 34 Working Group, 1990). What is lacking however, are helpful guidelines for training courses and perhaps more significantly the human and physical resources to run them. What we hope to do in this chapter is to discuss some of the issues that we have encountered as we have developed IT courses for nurses, and some of the lessons that we have learnt.

It is important to point out that this chapter assumes some knowledge of IT. It is written for the experienced teacher of IT and does not provide an adequate introduction to teaching IT for those with no background in this subject.

One way in which we have found it helpful to think about IT training, is in terms of a progressive or incremental model, see Fig. 6.1. This shows the progression from knowledge of computer components, operating systems and basic concepts of various programs through to understanding and using more complex software. It is possible to learn wordprocessing without a knowledge of the operating system, or for that matter, how computers work. However, when relatively simple problems arise, the user must call on technical support. This is neither effective nor efficient use of staff time. Basic building blocks have to be mastered in order to progress to more advanced or complex skills. The basic blocks are not necessarily easier to understand. For example, operating system concepts are some of the most difficult to grasp. Once mastered, however, they will enable students to tackle other computer concepts with a degree of insight. It is important therefore that students are introduced to the more complex skills involved in using an operating system prior to learning software packages, which are in some cases easier to master. We have called this the 'wise route', indicated in Fig. 6.1. and we recommend that students follow wise routes. Understanding is vital if students are to tackle problems, snarlups, and disasters which will inevitably occur outside the class.

This approach synthesises traditional learning with experiential learning. At the beginning of the course students require information about IT, and this is provided by the staff. Having this knowledge is only half of the story, however, students need to learn how to use it. Using their knowledge is where hands-on experiential learning plays its part. The aim is not only to produce people who can use IT, but to produce people who will know why they are using it, the principles behind IT, and the possibilities and problems of IT.

A STRUCTURED PROGRAMME OF LEARNING

There is a debate about how IT is best taught – whether it should be student or lecturer directed. Mark and Lange (1987), for example, concluded from their study of a graduate students' spreadsheet course that independent

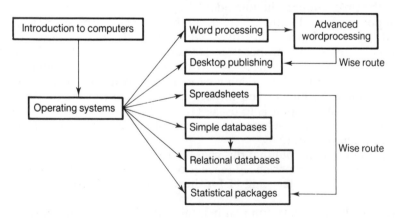

Fig. 6.1 Learning progression flow chart

learning, with the onus on the student to seek tutorial support, was not the best way to promote learning in this field. They recommend regular, scheduled, structured laboratory sessions. Tasks they state, should be demonstrated, then practised with supervision before being tried independently with help available if and when necessary. What is not clear from their study is the structure and content of the student learning manuals. It would seem that reappraisal of these 'tools' may have been needed before dismissing the student led approach entirely. We would agree that acquiring computing skills by distance learning requires a very high degree of motivation and commitment. However in our experience the student led approach can work very well provided the ground work is done and the student learning materials are carefully planned, piloted and constantly evaluated.

A core of packages has been developed by the Institute of Health Sciences, for a wide range of applications and ability levels. These have been developed with health service personnel in mind. Activities in nursing and health care that are computerised have been identified and simulations produced, to create as near reality situations as possible, in other words a practicum. Learning in this practicum, however, is also dependent on a degree of basic knowledge acquired from lecturing staff. In learning computing, there is no substitute for beginning at the beginning, obvious though that may seem!

Teaching strategies need to be sensitive to the student group. It is a mistake to assume skills in this particular subject area. There is a widespread belief that in the 1990s student nurses enter training with computer skills. An in-house questionnaire (100 student nurses) carried out during 1990 at a large teaching centre in Newcastle revealed that only 8% of respondents felt confident about their ability to use IT, and 42% reported no experience of computers or typewriting. Seniority does not guarantee IT proficiency either, and so there is also a need to make beginners' courses available to senior staff.

Introductory sessions

The introductory sessions are very important. If it is a beginners' course, then no computing knowledge must be assumed. Students, whether learners or qualified staff, need to be reminded that learning computing takes time and is seldom as simple as proficient users would have them believe. It takes time to learn new concepts (Childs, 1986; Rowntree, 1982) and skills; computing combines both of these. The introductory session should cover the following aspects

1. **What a computer actually is and what it can do.**
   This needs to be considered before persuading students of the potential benefits of the use of computers. Asking for definitions from the group is a useful starting point.

2. **The teacher needs to spend some time introducing students to computer components and their functions.**
   Some students suffer anxiety over the whereabouts of the on-off

switch! An actual computer is useful here, although slides or overhead transparencies could be used effectively. It is important to differentiate between input devices, the processing unit and RAM, output devices and ancillary storage devices. Students with IT skills will be able to demonstrate their knowledge during this session. The advantage of a classroom session is that larger numbers can be taught together.

3. **A discussion on the different types of programs available and their potential use in nursing.**
   The main applications – for example, spreadsheets, wordprocessing, databases, desktop publishing, statistical and graphics packages – can be introduced. This is where the teacher can again draw upon student knowledge within the group.

4. **The teacher needs to convey the importance of computer literacy amongst nurses.**
   This can be achieved by discussing the various ways in which IT is used in the Health Services, gearing this discussion to the experiences of the student group. This can be developed by asking nurses to solve a problem relevant to their practice, such as compiling a database of patients in order to monitor screening, or immunisations, a strategy used by Summers et al. (1990).

5. **The introductory session should allow students to ask questions about both the subject and their own anxieties.**
   If the environment is supportive and empathetic, students will be more likely to express their concerns.

6. **Having fun!**
   This can be the greatest ice breaker. There is an immense amount of commercially available software which is both easy and fun to use. Simple quizzes, health checks and keyboard skills programs can be used to introduce computer-naive students in a non-threatening way, to the technology. Being able to type is undoubtedly an advantage.

The introductory sessions should emphasise the challenge IT presents for nurses. As Prophit (1986) reminds us, the capabilities of the computer must be developed to facilitate and not replace the intelligent and sensitive qualities of the person. This applies to all areas of use, be they directly related to patient care or for administrative support. The quality of the effectiveness and efficiency in using computers will be determined entirely by the quality of the planners', developers' and users' thinking.

Learning packages

The packages each consist of User Manuals and computer files. They have been developed by academic staff within the institution. Some of the packages involved in-depth discussions with health care professionals. They are used by a wide range of students on the following courses:

1. Project 2000;

2. Diploma of Professional Studies in Nursing;
3. B.Sc(Hons) Nursing Science;
4. Postgraduate Diploma and M.Sc in Health and Social Research;
5. Certificate of Higher Education in Information Technology for Health Professionals;
6. Diploma of Professional Studies (Midwifery);
7. Post Graduate Certificate/Certificate of Education (Nursing and Midwifery);
8. B.Sc Nursing Studies/RN;
9. Introductory courses for health personnel from local Health Authorities and Family Health Services Authorities;
10. Specialist courses for Resource Management.

Before undertaking a detailed study of individual application packages some general points about their development need to be made. Manuals not only serve the student but they also serve the institution. To this end they become trade marks of that institution and therefore careful thought should go into a 'house style'. This is not necessarily arrived at immediately, but usually develops over time. Amendments are continually made in the light of experience.

The following are general guidelines that we have developed which may be of help to others who are thinking of developing learning packages and manuals for use by students:

1. Each component should be in a separate manual.
2. A list of learning outcomes should appear at the front of each manual, giving the student a clear idea of what it is they are expected to know and understand by the end of the component.
3. A contents page should be included giving clear guidance as to where various components appear.
4. An explanation of the application should be given in clear, easily understood terminology. Launching into creating a spreadsheet with reference to cells and formulae can only confuse and alienate those students who have neither seen nor heard of a spreadsheet. Diagrams and pictures are helpful here.
5. The instructions should be well spaced on the page, using a mixture of type faces for emphasis. Too much information on one page can be taxing even to the keenest of students.
6. Make use of diagrams, boxes and tables or screen dumps where possible. This not only conveys the message that software can be used to enhance text but also to facilitate the student's understanding.
7. Include self answered questions (SAQ) at frequent intervals. (Answers are given at the back of the book). This focuses the student's mind on the task completed and can draw on previously learnt aspects. It also allows the student to see the interconnectedness of the material.
8. Try out a small number of manuals on several groups of students before a large print run is ordered.
9. Make notes on a master copy of any problems the students have whilst using the manuals. This makes modifications at a later date much easier.

10. Keep the style friendly. Occasional comments such as 'relax those shoulders' or using comic names in databases can go a long way to ease tensions.
11. **BE AWARE OF TIME!** Writing student manuals, particularly those that require file creation (databases and spreadsheets) is a time consuming process. Teachers may need to have time off other duties in order to produce manuals of the standard and format required.

Packages have been produced to include:

1. Introduction to DOS;
2. Introduction to wordprocessing;
3. Intermediate and advanced wordprocessing;
4. Spreadsheets;
5. Simple and relational databases;
6. Statistical packages at beginner, intermediate and advanced levels;
7. Using CD-ROM.

To illustrate our approach we will concentrate on packages 1, 2, and 5.

1. Introduction to the disk operating system – DOS
This session follows on from the classroom introduction to the technology. Components of computers have been explained. For most students, learning DOS causes many conceptual problems. It is tempting to gloss over the functions of the operating system and go straight into applications. As the operating system underpins all other computer operations, it is wise to spend some time on the basic concepts. Knowledge of the start up procedure – 'booting' – is especially important to users. It is akin to starting a motorcar, it may be a simple matter of turning a key, but what if nothing happens? Those of us who know nothing about what goes on under the bonnet can only cry for help! With some knowledge we may at least check some basic connections.

Two hours teaching time on the basic concepts within DOS provides a useful and necessary foundation, this can then be built on throughout the applications modules when students save, retrieve, copy or delete their files. The learning outcomes, stated at the beginning of the manual, are listed in Fig. 6.2.

To facilitate learning, analogies are used wherever possible. For example, to understand the principles of file management, including the concepts of subdirectories and sub-subdirectories, a diagram of a large filing cabinet is used. 'Loose' or free files are immediately accessible on a shelf in the cabinet (i.e. no drawers to open). The subdirectories are the drawers and action must be taken (open drawer) before the contents (files) can be accessed.

Finding similarities between filenames, and students' own first and second names can also aid understanding. For example, the first filename (no more than eight letters) is descriptive, answering the question 'Who or what are you?' The extension name is a classification name answering the question 'To what family do you belong?' Thus the filename HEALTH.DOC implies that the file is about health (description) and is a document/text (family) file. Similarly the file CONFIG.SYS is a system (family) file concerned with the (description) computer set up (configuration). This approach to teaching concepts follows Bruner's (1977) theory that incoming information is related to a previously acquired frame of reference. Rowntree (1982) also supports the view that to enhance students' understanding of new concepts, model, counter and near examples should be considered. Thus the concept of a filing cabinet is frequently used to illustrate how the computer stores files.

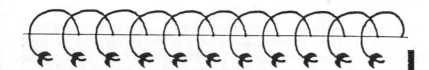

You will have mastered the basics of using DOS when you can:

- **_Boot_** your PC computer
- Check and change the **_time_** and **_date_** if necessary
- Establish the system **_default_** disk drive
- Obtain a **_list_** of a disk directory
- **_Format_** diskettes
- Understand file **_specifications_**
- **_Copy_** and **_delete_** files
- Organise and manage file **_subdirectories_**
- Start **_application_** programs

Fig. 6.2   MS-DOS Student Manual

During the DOS session students should have the opportunity of loading programs. It is also useful to put in the manual 'deliberate errors' so that students can become familiar with the computer's vocabulary. Terms such as Abort! Re-try! Cancel! can be rather worrying when met for the first time. This command can be induced by asking the computer to read the A: drive in which there is not a resident floppy. Exercises such as these can greatly increase the students confidence in using IT.

Wordprocessing package

This institution uses the business standard software Wordperfect[1] (at present version 5.1). This has been chosen as it is a very versatile program with advanced facilities. Students are provided with a keyboard template to assist the learning of commands. The help facility is excellent, following introductory sessions, motivated students can soon find out about the more complex functions within Wordperfect.

The wordprocessing sessions have been divided up into three main areas – introduction, intermediate and advanced. The objectives for each are indicated in Fig. 6.3.

Producing proficient typists is not our aim, therefore, text already typed is retrieved and the students edit, enhance and format this text. Wordperfect 5.1 is a sophisticated application with literally hundreds of commands.

Students should be encouraged to explore different uses for wordprocessing in their own field of work. Such exploration could include:

1. Producing assignments;
2. Producing posters and signs;
3. Creating memos or standard letter headings;
4. Producing diaries and off-duty sheets;
5. Care planning;
6. Setting up a 'mail merge' database of addresses in order to circulate newsletters or other information sheets.

Databases

This type of application is far more complex to learn than wordprocessing. It is better to proceed slowly, starting with the concepts of a database. Most students are familiar with a collection of records of one sort or another, using the principle of concept attainment discussed above, examples from the students' own experiences are used. The telephone directory is a fine example of a collection of records, as is card index system found in the library or the non-computerised doctor's surgery. Students are introduced to the database terminology: 'a record' – one case, which contains units of

---

[1] Wordperfect is a trademark of Wordperfect Corp. There are numerous texts to support the Wordperfect user from easy to read quick reference to more advanced texts.

information, which are referred to as 'fields' e.g. first name. The layout of the fields is referred to as a 'form'. Students can discuss the various ways a collection of records might be stored. For example, in the library record cards are stored by date, whereas other records may be stored in alphabetical order.

Understanding familiar concepts, students can then progress to the more complex principles of powerful electronic databases. Students are first

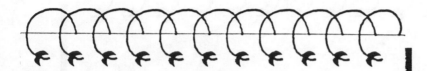

After this exercise students should know the basics of:

1. Loading Wordperfect 5.1
2. Starting the program and creating a document.
3. Entering text.
4. Saving and exiting.
5. Loading an existing file.
6. Cursor control for moving around the screen.
7. Copying, moving and deleting text.
8. Finding and replacing text.
9. Changing text.
10. Using help screens and menus.
11. Enhancing text.
12. Viewing and printing documents.

Fig. 6.3 Wordperfect 5.1. Student Introductory Manual

introduced to a simple database, using PCFILE (a public domain program selected for its cheapness and ease of use).

A minimum of four hours should be allowed to achieve the outcomes listed in Fig. 6.4.

Students then progress to more sophisticated programs such as dBASE IV.* This program has been chosen because it remains an established

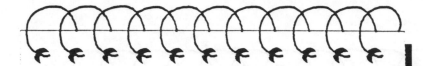

After this course students should know the basics of:

1. The differences between the field types: character, date, numeric and logic
2. Creating a simple database
3. Adding and deleting records
4. Finding records
5. Modifying records
6. Sorting the database
7. Changing the database definition
8. Writing letters and using mail merge
9. Producing reports

Fig. 6.4 PC-File Student Manual

---

*dBase IV is produced by Ashton Tate

standard, continued support is guaranteed and there is a vast amount of third party support, including books, and software that will read and manipulate dBASE files. Its programming capabilities (from its database management system base) also mean that it can be used to construct all kinds of applications.

Health service databases are of the relational variety, either as applications or 'master' databases. These systems usually use main frame technology. However with increasing power of PCs, adequate and appropriate starter skills can be learnt using, dBASE IV. Many health units and departments already have PC dBASE III or dBASE IV. Nurses will be expected to use these systems in hospitals and therefore need to have a working knowledge of them.

Introducing students to a simulation of a system, i.e. a relational database, Patient Administration System (PAS) has proved helpful before the students attempt the more advanced skill of creating their own relational database. The PAS application we use took several months to develop, and includes information on 100 patients admitted to two fictitious surgical wards during a one month period.

Students vary in their ability to learn how to use an application and go on to create a relational database. We have found that ten hours supportive tutoring can provide a firm foundation for most students (provided that they have the basic computing skills mentioned earlier).

An approach tried successfully is to set up 'deliberate errors'. The students can then see for themselves the result of inaccurately entered data. The object of the exercise is that the students must then go through the appropriate steps to put the record straight. This is one good way of understanding the importance of linking fields. If, for example, the wrong patient admission number is entered in the pathology department, the general practitioner (GP), if a fund holder, or the District Health Authority managing the GP of the actual patient whose admission number was used, will be billed for a test the patient did not have. The new contractual arrangements in the NHS require accurate accounting.

TEACHING IT

Who should teach IT?

The central issue here is whether nurses should develop expertise in and teach IT themselves, or 'call in' experts to do the job for them. There are advantages and disadvantages to both strategies. If nurses take on the teaching of IT they will develop their knowledge base, their skills and enhance their participation in the Health Service. One of the advantages of becoming part of higher education is the opportunity it offers to meet experts from other disciplines whose contribution can be considerable.

In practical terms, however, it is probably easier for nurses to do this teaching. Computer specialists cannot learn all there is to know about nursing in two months. In our experience, however, a nurse teacher in the same amount of time can develop a level of computer literacy which enables him or her to pass on these skills to students. It is not a question of learning all there is to know about computers, since the speed of the technological developments makes that an almost unattainable goal. Nor are nurse teachers expected to be programmers. Within our institution a compromise has been reached. Lecturers with an interest in IT who have a background in the social and health sciences (some of whom are also on the university register) have developed specialist IT skills. They have the use of polytechnic advanced computing facilities, including mainframe facitlities as well as the use of PC labs. This together with their knowledge and insight into health care issues puts them in a good position to teach IT. We believe that all teachers of IT to health care students should have:

1. A knowledge and understanding of the basic components of computer systems;
2. A knowledge and understanding of different types of computers;
3. A knowledge, understanding and ability to use a variety of applications for example wordprocessing, databases (simple and relational), spreadsheets and graphics packages and statistical programs;
4. A knowledge of the use, within the health care field, of various applications;
5. Knowledge of some of the wider issues associated with the use of IT – for example the Data Protection Act, health and safety issues and the effects of technological change on organisations.

Training for nurse teachers can be found in a variety of organisations. Commercial software companies offer short courses, and some institutions of higher and further education have established reputations in this field.

When and where should the teaching take place?

Timing the teaching of IT is important. Ideally, it should begin as student nurses start their education, but the reality is that there is a large number of nurses already qualified who do not have IT skills.

Wherever a nurse is in his or her career, the initial emphasis needs to be on gaining basic skills. The objectives of any basic skills course should be clearly stated, not only for teachers but also made available for the students. The myth that students are somehow better off by not knowing the expected learning outcomes is no longer tenable. Involving students from the very beginning in the learning process ensures that it is them rather than the teacher who decides whether or not the objectives have been met (Knowles 1984). This is particularly important in teaching computing. A student should be able to develop at his or her own pace, there is little sense in moving on to higher order skills or cognitive levels when learning at a lower level has not taken place. When a course on spreadsheets for graduate nurses was piloted in the United States, Mark and Lange (1987) found that without a basic knowledge of computers it proved very difficult for course participants to grasp the spreadsheet concepts and use the application effectively. The ideal, therefore, would be to implement a series of introductory sessions. End tests would be one way of assessing whether objectives had been met, but ultimately the student would be the best judge of his or her own learning, reflecting the andragogic ideology in contemporary nurse education (Knowles 1984).

It is impossible to lay down specific guidelines for the number of hours to be set aside for computer teaching within an undergraduate/pre-registration curriculum, although it is reasonable for minimum numbers of hours to be stated. One paper describing a basic computing course for nurse teachers, (Rafferty 1991) quotes 35 hours for each student, half of which is devoted to hands-on work. This amount of time is probably an unaffordable luxury in most undergraduate or training programmes. A minimum of ten hours, however, for each student during the first 18 months of training allows for reasonable understanding of the basic concepts. Two hours (which could be separated) of this time should be spent on discussing IT and its place in nursing and health care. This classroom based session helps to set the scene for the ensuing practicals and may go some way to convince the a reluctant student of the merits of learning IT. A further six hours (over and above the initial ten hours) during the branch programmes of a Project 2000 course or in final year of pre-Project 2000 courses, would offer reinforcement of and possible enhancement of the basic skills. Students from other post-registration or post graduate positions should be offered a similar number of hours training. The introductory sessions need to be close together to aid retention of newly acquired knowledge. Opportunities and facilities for students to practise in their own time should also be available.

The teaching of IT can be integrated with other subject areas, for instance, it could be discussed in nursing management, which could include care planning and allocation of resources; the research process; health policy and epidemiology. This emphasises the important and necessary links between computing and other disciplines. It must be stressed however that at this level we are aiming only to lay the foundation from which intermediate and advanced level skills can develop.

There are very few schools and colleges of nursing that boast a surfeit of rooms. In fact the contrary is often the case. Computing facilities to meet the proposed curriculum developments cannot be accommodated in an ad hoc fashion. Not only are special cabling and electrical entry points needed, but ergonomic issues must be considered. If proper attention is not paid to the planning of computing laboratories (lighting, spacing, swivel chairs) the quality of teaching will suffer.

Liaising with polytechnics and universities has increased the resources available to nurse teachers and students. Purpose built computer labs are now available for teaching sessions. Investment in such facilities by schools and colleges of nursing is much less costly than setting up an 'in-house' facility and students are usually willing to travel as they are now quite used to being taught in a variety of venues. Capital costs are not the only financial outlay when planning computing laboratories, maintenance and upgrading costs must also be considered. If a school decides to invest in its own facilities it should purchase the best machines it can afford, rather than being attracted to the cheapest available. This does not necessarily mean going for the most famous name, but being influenced by the power, speed and capacity of the PC itself.

In this institution we have laboratories with 16 PCs equipped with 386 processors, 40 megabyte hard disks and 3.5 inch floppy disk drives. MS-DOS versions 3.3 or 4.01 are installed on the machines. Several programs have been copied onto the individual hard disks, while other programs are offered via the university network.

As the technology within the health care systems (and elsewhere) moves away from huge centralised systems (one large processor and many 'dumb' terminals) to a more work station approach (stand alone machines with networking arrangements), learning can realistically take place on PCs. The skills learnt, while not necessarily immediately applicable to the usual main frame hospital environment, are transferable.

On-line printing facilities should be available, providing both wide continuous and single sheet feed services. If students are producing tables or graphs, then either dot matrix or laser facilities should be provided. Daisy wheel printers may produce fine letter quality print but cannot easily produce graphs. Institutions may need to look at printing costs per student, especially where laser printing is available. This should cause few problems as students are, in most instances, willing to pay for photocopying.

From experience it is clear that for learning outcomes to be achieved, each student must have his or her own machine during the teaching sessions. This should be the case for all levels of instruction.

Teacher/student ratios in computing courses needs to be higher than in most other areas. What also needs to be taken into account is the numbers of computer literate students already in the group. These students should be 'shared' between the groups and their experience and skills used to help their peers and the teacher. Carefully prepared, 'in-house' student manuals are invaluable here; not only can they meet the needs of the particular student group but they enable individuals to work at their own pace. Others, therefore, are not held back while the teacher is engaged in one to one support.

There has been a tendency to use commercially produced training tutorials. This tends to be counter productive as they invariably assume knowledge, are not customised and are often full of jargon.

CONCLUSION

The authors recognise that computers have become and will remain an integral part of health care. We believe that nurses should be introduced to the basic computing concepts at an undergraduate level i.e. during training, or for those already qualified, during post registration courses. Nurse teachers should be given every opportunity to gain or enhance their computing skills. First level courses should include basic information about the technology, computing concepts, knowledge of operating systems, wordprocessing, the principles of simple databases and spreadsheets and the use of CD-ROM. For this learning to be meaningful and relatively permanent, students must have hands-on experience. There is value in classroom teaching in order to consider the implications of the use of technology in nursing, but there is no substitute for practical sessions. For those nurses who have attained a basic competency, opportunities should be made available for them to develop those skills further. This may reasonably be as a chosen option rather than a statutory requirement. Specialised IT courses can be developed that explore the use of spreadsheet, statistics and database applications in the practice of nursing. This could be in research, nurse management, clinical areas and education.

This latter area includes not only pre-registration and post-registration education, but also patient education. Firby et al. (1991) report on a recent initiative to introduce CAL into patient education. It seems all areas of health care are harnessing the computer technologies. Their study, although in an area still in its infancy, supports the now indisputable view that for new computer initiatives to succeed, the staff involved must feel comfortable and competent with the technology. From her study of nurses' attitudes towards computerisation, Sultana (1990) recommends that computer-orientation courses be made part of the all education and training programmes for nurses. A positive attitude can be developed through knowledge and understanding of the subject.

Specialist courses in IT are being developed across the country. The University of Northumbria at Newcastle launched a Certificate of Higher Education in Information Technology Course for Health Professionals. This modular part-time, one-year course offers 72 hours practical computing; 24 hours studying the impact of technology on the individual, the organisation and society; 24 hours visiting and discussing applications of IT and 60 hours devoted to a project which includes the development of an application for use in an area of health care. As a development from this course, we hope to offer a Diploma in IT and a health informatics branch within our M.Sc programme.

We are also able to offer short, introductory and specialist courses for health service personnel. The timing of these courses has been tailored to meet the needs of the students attending.

Attention must be given to the production of student learning materials. These not only provide the instructions for a particular session but should become part of a long term resource package. Teachers should be given the opportunity to enhance their computing skills from time to time, in order to keep pace with new developments. Visits to various sites within and without health service areas can stimulate and encourage motivation as well as giving insight into the varied uses of IT.

Nurses are expected to be innovators in the field of health care. Information technology represents a major innovation. Proficiency in IT offers nurses the opportunity to use this development as a means for finding new and better ways to deliver care.

REFERENCES

Bruner, J.S. (1974) *Towards a Theory of Instruction*. Harvard University Press, Cambridge, MA.

Chambers, M. and Coates, V.C. (1990) Computer training in nurse education: a bird's eye view across the UK. *Journal of Advanced Nursing.* **15**, 16–21.

Childs, D. (1986) *Psychology and the Teacher*, 4th edition. Cassell, London.

DoH (1990) *Framework for Information Systems: Overview.* Working Paper 11, HMSO, London.

Firby, P.A., Luker, K.A., Caress, A.L. (1991) Nurses' opinions of computer-assisted learning for use in patient education. *Journal of Advanced Nursing*, **16**, 987–95.

Knowles, M. (1984) *The Adult Learner: A Neglected Species*. Gulf Publishing Co., London and Houston.

Mark, B.A. and Lange, L. (1987) Spreadsheets in nursing administration. Not as easy as 1-2-3. *Computers in Nursing.* **5 (6)**, 214–18.

Prophit, P. (1987) Introductory Chapter in *Computers and their Applications in Nursing*. Lippincott, London and Philadelphia.

Rafferty, T. (1991) Teaching teachers. *British Journal of Health Care Computing.* **May**, 17–18

Rowntree, D. (1982) *Educational Technology in Curriculum Development*. Harper and Row, London.

Sultana, N. (1990) Nurses' attitudes towards computerisation in clinical practice. *Journal of Advanced Nursing*, **15**, 696–702.

Summers, S., Penny, S., Fortin-Boyer J., Loutzenhiser, J. and Arnold-Biagioli B. (1990) Creative use of microcomputer software by graduate student nurses. *Computers in Nursing.* **8 (5)** 198–200.

Section Three
Practicums

Introduction

The teaching strategies in this section are somewhere in the middle of the continuum that we described in our introduction. They involve addressing basic knowledge, but they also involve coaching students through the problems and issues that they face in practice by using practicums. The Interpersonal Communication Skills (IPCS) strategy (Chapter Seven) sets up a practicum using closed circuit television, in which students can explore practice issues in the presence of a coach or teacher. This involves role plays, which the students write themselves, thus ensuring that they have control over the content of the sessions. The strategy also involves the use of a workbook which students complete, and which requires them to summarise basic concepts in communication theory. From this workbook they extract the theoretical basis of their role play. Perhaps the most important part of the IPCS course is the discussions that take place after the role plays, in which teachers and students begin to evaluate the theory using practice as a yardstick. Here, practice issues, either actual or possible, are presented, and the ability of the theoretical literature to address them is discussed. Students often use these sessions to rehearse potential issues that they may face, or to re-examine experiences that they have had, and the role of the teacher is to suggest as many different ways of looking at a problem as possible.

In Chapter Eight, which is about teaching research methods, a similar process occurs. The practicum is of essential importance here, as it may be the only opportunity students have to experience taking part in a research project. Here the teaching sessions do not necessarily correspond to real life as the students daily experience it, but it is anticipatory, in that one day they may wish to do research of their own. However, because of the students' lack of knowledge about the world of the research project, this imposes a more directive approach on the teacher. Issues such as ethical committees, the practicalities of data collection, and the problems that can occur in even the most straightforward project, need to be carefully controlled by the teacher.

An interesting point about these strategies is that when in the role of coach, the teacher often seems to be much more pragmatic than the students. It is often the teacher that points out that the texts are idealistic or impractical, or that they do not consider other issues that may affect practice. Students tend to be over-awed by texts, and over-critical of practice, and often make quite simplistic decisions about what should be done. Teachers therefore have to point out the problems with this, drawing upon their own experience, and the knowledge they have of students' experiences. In doing this, the teacher is acting as a role model, and demonstrating how theory can be used and developed in practice.

7 Teaching interpersonal communication skills

Jan Reed

INTRODUCTION

Within nursing there has been a degree of disquiet expressed about the communication skills of nurses. Bridge and Macleod Clark (1981) for example, write in their foreword that the research evidence they present about communication skills in nursing shows the nature of nurse-patient communication to be 'both disturbing and unsatisfactory'. Nurses in their view, and in the view of many of the contributors to their book, are not skilled in communication, with a number of serious consequences for patient care. Poor communication, particularly poor information giving, is a major concern for patients, as a number of researchers have demonstrated (see May 1990 for an overview). In addition, there is an argument that good communication has potential therapeutic effects, which are not fully appreciated in nursing practice. The work of Hayward (1975), for example, indicates that information about surgical procedures, can reduce post-operative pain, as measured by requests for analgesia.

In addition to these reported effects of communication, the nurse-patient relationship is becoming of central importance to current discussions of nursing. As nursing develops values of holistic individualised care, this demands a greater emphasis on the psychological aspects of nursing. If the patient is viewed holistically, then this view, by definition, must address the issues of anxiety, stress, self-esteem, and a myriad of non-physiological aspects of care. Similarly, individualised care cannot be conducted without careful assessment, evaluation, and negotiation with the patient, all of which demand communication skills.

Given that most of the research on communication skills in nursing indicates deficiencies, and that communication is seen to be increasingly important, this suggests a need for more education for nurses (Kagan 1985). Educational input in this area has, in the past, been conspicuous by its absence, as Gott (1983) discovered in her research. This study looked at many areas of nurse education, testing the hypothesis that 'training schools do not prepare student nurses adequately for work experience'. This hypothesis was supported by the research, but in addition the students in the study also highlighted their perceived lack of preparation for communication with patients. This was supported by observation data which examined their communication skills, with only 15% being judged by the researchers to be 'facilitative to the communication process' (Gott 1983: p.123).

Sweeping recommendations for 'more education' are, however, based upon the assumption that these skills can be taught and operationalised without too many problems, an assumption that would be challenged by anyone who has attempted to mount a programme of this type. Part of the problem is that the criticisms of communication skills are mainly of an individualistic nature, in that 'good' communication is seen as a property or characteristic of an individual, and is unrelated to the wider social arena in which the communication takes place. This perspective ignores the many environmental, cultural, and practical problems that arise in communication, problems that are difficult to incorporate into a training programme.

This focus on teaching communication skills in a decontextualised way can lead to a procedural approach, in other words that skills can be reduced to a series of steps (rather like ballroom dancing). The initial greeting of a patient to the ward, for example, could be broken down to a series of gestures and phrases, which could be rehearsed until proficiency was achieved. The student could then be expected to carry out this procedure whenever required.

This approach does, however, raise a number of issues about the degree to which such rule-governed behaviour would be seen as empathetic or genuine by the patient, whether it would foster individualised care, and whether it is actually possible to learn enough procedures to encompass all clinical events. These questions would suggest that what is needed is a more flexible approach, which would enable students to develop understanding and insight into communication issues, and be able to evaluate and develop their skills in a variety of clinical situations.

This insight can be developed in part, by reading research and theory in the field of communication. There is a danger, however, that this research can be interpreted as definitive instructions for practice. Much of this research, in particular that derived from psychology, with a laboratory based, experimental approach, has of necessity a very narrow focus, which does not incorporate the myriad complexities of real life situations. Even research which is based in the field, including nursing research, has limitations in the way it addresses the place of communication alongside other aspects of patient care. It is extremely difficult to examine communication in nursing in a way which captures the complexities of practice, yet research which does not encompass these complexities becomes decontextualised and difficult to apply to practice.

Using this research as prescriptions for care is to court the problems inherent in the 'technical rationality' model of professional knowledge described by Schon (1987), and in so doing limit the development of reflective practice. The strategy chosen, therefore, was to attempt to develop a practicum, with the lecturer taking on a coaching role. In itself, however, this practicum, was insufficient; students could not draw upon theory unless they developed some knowledge of what this was, and so the IPCS course also had to provide a means of students understanding this body of theory.

TEACHING STRATEGY

With these thoughts in mind, a two-part strategy was devised in order to address the teaching of interpersonal communication skills to nurses, comprising a library-based, self-directed learning package and a programme of related group exercises. In this way it was hoped that students would not only develop information retrieval and analysis skills, but also develop the skills of critically applying such information and theory to practice. In the group exercises students would use their reading as a basis for the activities, but would be able to develop an understanding of how these could relate to practice issues through the discussions and role plays.

The workbook

The learning package has three sections. The first section asks students to make notes about a variety of concepts which are basic to an understanding of communication (such as verbal and non-verbal communication), with the instruction that they will draw upon a variety of theoretical and research texts and journal articles to complete this section. The second section asks students to review a number of nursing research articles about communication, and the third section asks them to observe and record a nurse-patient interaction.

This structure is designed to foster a progressive development of analytic ability in the students. The first section, where students are asked to summarise a variety of concepts and terms, is designed to consolidate their information retrieval skills. Students are asked to summarise concisely these concepts in a way that clearly demonstrates their understanding. They are not, at this stage, asked to be critical of the reading they have done, simply to communicate their understanding of the key concepts. The research review section continues this theme of concise summary by requiring students to describe, within a short word limit, a number of research studies. This is then developed by asking them to write a much more lengthy research review of a particular piece of research, in which they are able to be more critical.

The final section, the record of a nurse-patient interaction, returns them to 'real life', by focusing on an actual event in the context in which it took place. In this section they are able to draw upon literature they have read to analyse this interaction, but another intention is to develop their powers of observation. It is expected that they select interactions involving other nurses rather than themselves, so the opportunities for self-reflection are limited, but the process of reflecting on someone else's practice has value in that it can indicate to students how they may reflect upon their own.

Groupwork

The programme of group exercises is based on the use of closed circuit television (CCTV) facilities. After some initial warm up exercises, which acclimatise the group to the studios and the dreaded experience of seeing themselves on video, the class is divided into small groups and asked to write their own role plays to explore a selection of concepts covered in the workbook. There is a degree of freedom in the format of the role plays, in that students can focus on a very narrow aspect of the concept, or take a wider view, but they are asked to try to use events from practice as a basis for the role plays. In addition to the role plays, a workshop is held which centres on the observations of nurse-patient interactions they had recorded, in which they are asked to identify and discuss the relevance of the theoretical reading that they had done to the practice they had observed.

The programme of group exercises is intended to create, as far as possible, a practicum (Schon 1987) in which students could enter a 'virtual world', and in which they could explore practice issues. The extent to which this succeeds, however, is debatable, given the obvious differences between the CCTV studio and the clinical areas. Apart from the environmental differences (the studio is essentially a room with some chairs and thick curtains) the presence of the CCTV cameras is certainly a major difference between the studio and practice areas. Surprisingly, however, most students do become comfortable with the cameras after a few sessions, although some students did not participate as much as others. Participation is not enforced, as it is felt that this would be an insensitive and disrespectful invasion of their rights as students, but it is debatable whether these students gain as much from the programme as those who participate more fully.

Allowing the students to write their own role plays, which draw upon their clinical experience, is a strategy designed to maximise the potential for students to reflect on practice. Similarly, the group discussion after the role plays is focused on the extent to which these incidents had been experienced throughout the group, and the strategies students had used, or had seen others use to deal with them. Discussion is also encouraged about other possible scenarios, along the lines of 'what do you think would have happened if the nurse/patient had not done that?'

This strategy is used to allow students to experience reflection *on* practice (i.e. the retrospective analysis of behaviour at some time after it has occurred). This is not reflection *in* practice, which is the process which practitioners go through during their activities. It is, however, a step towards the development of this skill. The use of role plays which have a semi-fictional status, and can be about others, is similarly a step towards reflective practice, rather than reflection itself. It allows issues to be tackled in a way which is not threatening, and in which there is little pressure for self-validation or justification.

There was a degree of apprehension among the staff about the dangers of using role plays. Concerns were expressed about the ability of students to 'come out' of role, and the possibility that students could raise issues that would distress themselves or others. Care was taken therefore, to give the students clear guidelines about role play, and the discussion afterwards was handled in a way that would encourage dissociation from the roles that had been played. For example, at the end of play-back lecturers or students would joke, or sometimes applaud, as a way of marking the end of the role play. Discussion afterwards was couched in impersonal terms – for example, referring to the characters as 'the patient' rather than by the student's name. This appeared successful in that no students continued the role after the role play, and were able to talk about the role they had played in the same way as other members of the group.

The role plays did not appear to arouse any feelings of distress in the student group, perhaps because the students themselves did not choose topics, such as terminal care, which would arouse these feelings. The fact that they steered clear of very emotive issues could be regarded as a weakness in the programme, in that the issues chosen were possibly superficial. This was their choice, however, and it is difficult to see how one could coerce students into tackling issues in a way that they feel is inappropriate. The group work was directed by two members of staff, partly to facilitate group feedback and direct discussion, but also in case it became necessary for one lecturer to support a distressed student while the rest of the group carried on the discussion. This has not happened, but it would appear to be a sensible precaution to have two members of staff available for this type of work.

THE GROUPS

This package has been used with two different groups. Initially it was used with the DPSN (part time registered nurses), and later adapted for use with the BSc (Hons) Nursing Studies students (pre-registration students). There were significant differences in the way that these groups took part in the exercise. The DPSN appeared initially to be much more anxious about the CCTV, and expressed much more hostility to the idea of needing any coaching in this area. One student very angrily asserted that it was a waste of time 'because if we haven't got good skills by now, it's a waste of time doing anything about it'. This is a fair point to make, in that experienced nurses have developed strategies of communication over a long period of time, and a few hours of CCTV work is unlikely to revolutionise their approaches. Changing approaches, however, was not necessarily the object of the exercise, it was rather to encourage and facilitate a closer analysis of their practice, which could well involve a clearer appreciation of their skills, as much as their deficits. The points made by the students were acknowledged, therefore, and the lecturers stressed that they would not be 'teaching' skills, but allowing the students to develop their existing insights and abilities.

The pre-registration students were mystified by the idea of communication skills; their experience of practice was so limited that they had no clear idea of what nurses' work involved, still less of the issues that could arise from communication with patients. They were, however, less inhibited about the CCTV, and generally ready to 'have a go' at anything.

The scenarios chosen by the two groups for their role plays differed considerably. Whereas the DPSN chose incidents from their practice, the pre-registration students did not have this experience to draw upon. They therefore tended to choose GP/patient interactions, probably because this represented the area in which they had most experience of health care.

There was, however, a potential problem, in that this scenario was difficult to link to nursing practice, and therefore the lecturers had to work extremely hard to pick out issues and apply them to possible incidents in nursing. Thus where, for example, a role play explored the ways in which the social class of a patient could affect a GP's manner, the lecturers had to turn the discussion to ways in which it could affect nurses' perceptions. As most of the portrayals of GPs were negative, it was felt important to emphasise that doctors are not the only 'bad guys', and that nurses are equally likely to be rude, unpleasant or insensitive.

Negative portrayals were common in both student groups, i.e. examples of 'bad' communication skills were presented more than 'good'. There are several possible reasons for this. Firstly this type of role play is easier to write and more vivid to perform – supportive communication is much more low key. Secondly, close relationships are seen as taking time to develop, something which cannot be portrayed in a five-minute role play. Thirdly, the students were embarrassed about acting roles which were 'sickly sweet' in front of their peers, although they may adopt this approach in practice. The use of negative examples was discussed in the group sessions, and this provided some interesting debates. The embarrassment at being seen as 'too sweet', was particularly interesting, as the students came to the conclusion that they would be seen as 'traitors' to other nurses, particularly if the patient was generally unpopular. This dividing the world into 'us' (nurses) and 'them' (patients) was explored further, and lead to discussions of literature, for example Menzies (1960), which discusses defence mechanisms in nursing. The issue was not resolved in the group discussions, but they had offered students a different way of thinking about their practice.

ASSESSMENT

The IPCS workbook is a formally assessed piece of work, which students must pass. As such it is subject to the same marking criteria as all other pieces of academic work. These criteria, however, do assume a degree of student responsibility for structuring written work, which is part of the process of writing essays or projects. In the IPCS workbook, however, the structure is largely determined by the lecturers, in that the sections to be completed are very much self-contained, and clearly specified. Using criteria such as 'organisation of material' is clearly not appropriate for this assignment. Additional criteria then had to be developed for this particular assignment, and clarify the difference between levels of analysis. These criteria focused on the skills of summary and clarity of communication, and breadth of reading. An excellent submission would therefore be one in which the student had used a wide variety of material, summarised and evaluated it concisely, and given clear indication of their understanding of the topic. A poor submission would be one in which the student had used a narrow range of material, drawing upon a limited number of sources, had been unable to present their summary concisely, had done so in an uncritical way, and indicated that the student did not understand the concept in question. (A copy of these criteria is given in Fig. 7.1)

The quality of student work varied, as expected, with marks ranging from 35% (fail) to 80% (first class). Those at the lower end of the scale were students who had attempted to complete the workbook without using any reference material. These therefore tended to be anecdotal and, on occasion, self-contradictory. These students tended to write in an unfocused way, and not only was their work rambling, but it was also difficult to relate it to the topic heading.

The middle band of students, those achieving between 50% and 60%, were those who had produced thorough pieces of work, but which did not move beyond the purely descriptive. Although they met the criteria for brevity, they did not produce work which met the criteria for a high mark. The students who did went beyond this basic level, comparing and contrasting theories and research, relating the sections of the workbook

---

The following guidelines should be used when marking the IPCS workbooks. No relative weighting is given to the sections, and the mark should be expressed in a percentage (i.e. out of 100%).

Concepts of communication

Where the student has been asked to summarise concepts of communication, it is expected that this should draw upon a range of literature, both discursive and research based, nursing and non-nursing. The student should **concisely** and **clearly** summarise the concept in a way that indicates their understanding, and should show the ability to differentiate between types of literature used. Students who write at length, or to no great purpose should be penalised. At this stage students are not expected to have developed sophisticated critical analytic skills, but those who do demonstrate a level of understanding beyond the descriptive should be rewarded.

CCTV Exercises

Here the students have been asked to write up the CCTV exercises. The first two exercises, 'the balloon game' and 'hidden agendas' are **not** assessed, they were only to acclimatise the students to CCTV. In the other exercises, however, students are assessed on their ability to **clearly** and **concisely** describe the exercise. They may choose to write up only their own group work, or both group exercises in the session. These sections do not rely on references, but students who do use references should be rewarded.

Research reviews

Here students are asked to **summarise** 5 studies, and review one further study in greater depth. All reviews should contain enough pertinent information for the reader to determine the methods and results of the research. Those reviews which do not include this type of detail, or any details which would confirm that the paper was empirical research, should be penalised. In the longer review, students are not expected to critique methodology etc in any depth, but those student who do evaluate the research, compare it to other studies, or discuss the relevance to practice should be rewarded.

Fig 7.1

to each other, and relating their written work to clinical practice, often using literature outside the field of communication. These students also demonstrated a use of references outside the field of nursing, i.e. rather than relying on 'potted versions' of communication theory, specially written for nursing, they went to the original work in social psychology.

Overall the work was well done, and at a level expected at the stage of the student's course, either DPSN or BSc (Hons). The skills developed in a previous assignment, an information retrieval skills package, were reinforced, and students showed signs of beginning to relate theory to practice. This was often done in a simplistic and prescriptive way, however, with students making statements such as 'the nurse must accept the cultural differences of the patient'.

Some of the most interesting parts of the workbook were the sections where the students had written up the group exercises. Some had merely recounted events, whereas some had related the exercises to theoretical and/or clinical issues. Some students had used these sections to discuss events in practice, or to describe the changes in their thinking that had resulted from the exercises. Fascinatingly, each student's account was completely individual, with a number coming to completely different conclusions.

EVALUATION

The IPCS course was evaluated in terms of student perception rather than behavioural change. Behavioural change was impossible to identify in either group, without vast resources, and additionally implies a simple causal relationship between teaching and behaviour, which is extremely dubious. The DPSN group were asked for anonymous comments on the IPCS component, as part of the overall course evaluation. This produced a limited amount of feedback which, although it was generally positive, did not allow us to develop the component very much.

The comments that we did receive were typically about initially feeling uncomfortable about CCTV, but adjusting to it as the course progressed. Some students did find that it had been more useful than expected, and had given them more confidence and understanding, but there were a number who had felt that the usefulness was limited. These students also commented that they had taken part in similar exercises and courses before, and so they felt that they were repeating previous learning. These students were in the minority, but it may well be the case that their proportions increase as pre- and post-registration education uses similar methods more frequently. If this is the case, then it will not necessarily mean that we can treat such learning as the norm, but it does mean that we will have to be careful that we allow students to extend their knowledge and understanding, rather than make them cover the same ground again. One possible strategy is to use these students' prior experience more explicitly in discussion sessions, and perhaps giving them a clear role in leading groupwork. With the minimal amount of information we obtained from the questionnaire, however, it was difficult to draw any conclusions other than that most students had enjoyed the experience.

Because of the limitations of the DPSN evaluation strategy, a different approach was developed for the undergraduate group, using a variation of nominal group technique (Delbecq 1975) which took place in a formal session. Nominal group technique is extensively used in a variety of educational and training sessions, and can be used to evaluate entire programmes or components of programmes. Evaluating components is perhaps more manageable, and the evaluation can be very focused, whereas whole course evaluation can become embroiled in a number of issues, such as catering facilities, which are not particularly useful.

Using nominal group technique is a way of collating individual responses to develop a profile of the group response, which is difficult to achieve when qualitative comments are collected. Nominal group technique does not convert qualitative comments into numerical values, but it does provide a ranking system for the issues raised. Another advantage of this approach is that it also generates positive comments, whereas some evaluation strategies can bias responses towards the negative, in that problems are often more easily identified than successes.

The form of nominal group technique used in this evaluation was a focused and polarised one. The group were asked to focus on the IPCS component, as opposed to any other part of the course, and were asked to think of positive and negative aspects. The session started with each student in turn being asked to think of one positive aspect of the IPCS course, and to shout it out to the staff member who was given the job of recording the responses on the whiteboard. When no new comments were made, the exercise was stopped. The same procedure was repeated asking for negative aspects to be identified, and again, when this category was saturated, the exercise stopped. The lists of negative and positive categories were then discussed to determine whether any comments should be collapsed, because they were repetitious, or expanded because they did not cover the points the students wished to make. Having finalised the lists, the students were then asked to write down their individual ranking for the points identified. These were then collected by staff and analysed. The results are summarised in Fig. 7.2.

Positive points	Negative points
1. Made you think about yourself	1. CCTV embarrassing
2. Increased your confidence	2. Didn't always know enough about nursing to write role plays
3. Let you discuss things that worried you about nursing	3. Workbook involved a lot of time
4. CCTV was good fun, not boring lectures	4. Some people didn't join in CCTV work
5. You were allowed to choose your own role plays – didn't feel controlled by lecturers	5. Didn't appreciate some of it until on the wards

Fig. 7.2   BSc (Hons) Nursing Studies IPCS Evaluation

Only the first five points in each category are given in Fig. 7.2, as beyond this the ranking scores were negligible, and in fact there were only five points raised on the negative side. It is interesting to note that conflicting comments were made about the CCTV (i.e. that it was both fun and embarrassing). This technique allows you to identify opposing perceptions like this, which in other forms of evaluation may result in marks cancelling out and a neutral score being given.

Another interesting point is that although confidence building was high on the list of positive points, it was not the positive aspect ranked highest. This was 'making you think' which is an encouraging finding, in that students seemed to find this the most important aspect of the teaching. The student comments also indicate that they appreciated the style of the sessions, in that they felt that they had a degree of control and ownership of the work done. The informal presentation of the sessions was felt to allow a number of 'incidental' issues to be discussed.

The negative points were largely expected, indeed the discomfort felt about CCTV had been predicted by the staff, in fact we were more surprised that this had been also identified as 'fun'. The comments about 'not knowing enough about nursing' when writing role plays does demand some reconsideration of the IPCS component. Students obviously felt that their knowledge did not always enable them to make their role plays realistic, and they certainly contained inaccurate details and some rather peculiar medical terms. The role plays did, however, demonstrate a degree of emotional validity, in that the scenarios chosen did reflect some realistic interpersonal behaviours. The component could possibly be run later in the course, but this would then lose the advantage of preparing students for practice, which was highlighted in the second evaluation strategy.

This was a semi-structured questionnaire that students completed away from the class, and returned anonymously to staff. In it they were asked to record any comments they wished to make about the IPCS component. This was structured in a broadly narrative way – i.e. the students were asked to record how they felt about communication skills before, during, and after the course. This strategy was used to 'flesh out' the comments made in the evaluation session, in that it allowed students to make more detailed comments. As it was anonymous, it avoided the potential problem of peer group and staff influence determining responses, a potential problem in the group session. This strategy also allowed an overall evaluation of the component, which is problematic in the nominal group technique strategy. It does create a number of problems of data analysis, in that lengthy comments are often difficult to code and synthesise.

The data collected, however, did provide a vivid picture of the students perceptions in a way that the nominal group technique did not. The nominal group technique described consensus, whereas the qualitative questionnaire described individual variation (Quinn Patton 1990). An example of one of the comments was:

'At the time I thought it was just a laugh, but now I'm on the wards things from the IPCS keep flashing back, and I think 'Oh yes we talked about that'. My problem was that I didn't know enough about nursing to realise how important it was'.

Another student said:

> 'I did think it was ridiculous, teaching us to talk to people, I thought that it would produce insincere interactions. When the course started, however, I was reassured that you weren't going to try to give us scripts'.

These comments indicate a change of perception in the students as the course progressed, from suspicion and dismissal, to a higher valuation of the IPCS input. Perhaps the most interesting comment came from this student:

> 'I didn't realise there was so much to communication skills, and I went into the course feeling confident, and came out of it feeling terrified!'

In this case increased knowledge does not appear to have increased confidence, in fact the reverse would appear to be true. The aim of the IPCS component was not, however, primarily to increase confidence, but to stimulate reflection, and this does appear to have occurred. This student will need support in the clinical environment, though, if she is to relax and evaluate her interactions clearly.

Most of the comments made in the questionnaire were broadly positive, with the few negative comments which were made relating to the stress of CCTV. In this the results of this evaluation coincided with that of the DPSN. One student pointed out that the staff had not 'been made fools of' as the students had. This suggests that this student had not felt a sense of ownership in the work, and felt she had been coerced into participation. This was not the case, and the staff had, at the beginning of the course, offered their services in playing roles in the CCTV exercises, and were rather disappointed that they had not been accepted. To have forced staff into the groups would potentially have disrupted the work, and reduced student ownership.

Other negative comments concerned the timing of the component. A small number of students felt that they would have benefitted from more clinical experience first. This was contradicted by the other students who felt that it had been extremely useful preparation for ward work, not only in increasing skills and awareness, but in allowing them to 'rehearse' potential problems. One student has raised the issue of sexual harassment in one session, asking the lecturers advice about how she should deal with this. Others have asked questions about telling patients that they are dying, relatives becoming abusive, and a whole host of anticipated issues. These were discussed in the group by proposing possible strategies, proposals coming from staff and students, and so afforded opportunities for the group to work through some issues in a safe environment. The majority of comments about the timing of the sessions supported the view that they occurred in the right point in the course, although some students appeared concerned about this input ending:

> 'I suppose we're on our own now. What are we going to do when we need help in the future?'

CONCLUSION

The undergraduate students' comments indicate that the IPCS programme was a valued part of their preparation for practice, despite the initial anxieties about CCTV work. Interestingly some students, without prompting from staff, have actually made a video to show new applicants to the course, which suggests that for some at least, their terror was tinged with pleasure. In terms of the overall aims of the course, which was to develop self-awareness and reflective skills, the students' comments from both evaluation strategies suggest that this was achieved.

At this point, however, the long-term implications of the course cannot be evaluated, and there is a possibility, also identified by the students, that the benefits of this input may be lost if it is not consolidated in the clinical environment, and developed further in the course. The intention is to extend the IPCS component into the rest of the course, designing it to reflect the clinical experiences and concerns of the students. For example, when the students begin their second year they will have a mental health placement, and the IPCS workbook and group sessions will relate to models of counselling. Similarly in their third year, when they are increasingly aware of management issues, the IPCS will deal with organisational communication. In this way it is hoped to develop the students' awareness of communication skills in an appropriate and relevant manner.

All this will, of course, have limited effectiveness if the clinical experiences of the students do not also allow them to develop. This is dependent on the clinical settings and the staff there, particularly the mentors. In addition these students need support from their personal supervisors and the rest of the staff teaching them if they are to continue to increase their reflective skills, and their interpersonal awareness.

REFERENCES

Bridge, W. and Macleod Clark, J. (1981) *Communication in Nursing Care*. HM+M, London.

Delbecq, A.L. (1975) *Group Techniques for Program Planning*. Scott, Foreman and Co., Glenview.

Gott, M. (1983) *The Student Nurse: Initial Preparation and Performance*. Unpublished PhD thesis, Hull University.

Hayward, J. (1975) *Information: A Prescription Against Pain*. RCN, London.

Kagan, C.M. (ed.) (1985) *Interpersonal Skills in Nursing*. Croom Helm, London.

May, C. (1990) Research on nurse-patient relationships: problems of theory, problems of practice. *Journal of Advanced Nursing* **15**, 307–15.

Melia, K.M. (1982) 'Tell it as it is' – Qualitative methodology and nursing research: Understanding the student nurse's world. *Journal of Advanced Nursing* **7**, 327–35.

Menzies, I.E.P. (1960) *The functioning of Social systems as a defence against anxiety*. Tavistock Institute of Human Relations,

Quinn Patton, M. (1990) *Qualitative Evaluation and Research Methods*, 2nd ed. Sage Publications,

Royal College of Nursing (1982) *Research Mindedness in Nurse Education*. RCN, London.

Schon, D. (1987) *Educating the Reflective Practitioner*. Jossey-Bass, California.

8 Teaching research methods

Jan Reed and Susan Procter

INTRODUCTION

There is currently a movement in nursing to incorporate research methods into more and more nursing courses – not simply to enable nurses to evaluate research critically, but with the intention of enabling them to carry out research projects. As a result a growing number of courses require students to complete a research project as part of the course. This development can be related to some of the debates covered in the introductory chapters, in particular the increased professional status of nursing. Given that professional status is seen as partly dependent on a body of knowledge unique to nursing, it follows that nurses need to acquire the skills which will enable them to develop this. A further impetus for nurses to acquire skills in research methods is the current emphasis on quality assurance and service evaluation. These are primarily based on data collection and analysis which utilises similar skills to those developed in relation to research methods. This reinforces the importance of this subject on the nursing curriculum.

There are, however, some problems involved in developing research skills in nurses. The discussion in Chapter 2 highlighted the wide variety of methodologies currently utilised in nursing research. These range from the classical experimental method through epidemiology and survey research to ethnomethodology, phenomenology, grounded theory and into action research. Each of these approaches has a different history, different philosophy, and different criteria and objectives. To do justice to each of these methods demands a great deal of time and effort.

In addition to tackling these theoretical issues, there are a number of pragmatic issues which must be confronted when attempting to conduct a research project. Questions of time and resources are important, as are factors such as ethics committees and health authority policies which take time to negotiate. Given these problems, it is not surprising that where a research project forms only a small part of the course, the temptation is to direct students towards very small-scale studies, with limited theoretical and methodological discussion. As a result students' understanding and experience of research is limited to a very narrow and focused perspective which cannot hope to address the wide variety of methods that are potentially available to nurses.

It is important not to under-estimate the time and resources required to conduct even a small-scale study. Experience in teaching students on the Post-Graduate Diploma in Health and Social Research and the MSc in Health and Social Research suggest that even on courses which are primarily devoted to teaching research methods a number of students struggle to meet the deadlines often for reasons associated with the time it takes to gain access, then collect and analyse the data. On many nursing courses research methods are only one aspect of a much wider syllabus. If, as part of this course, students are expected to conduct a research study, the problems of data collection can overwhelm the project leaving students with insufficient time to develop their understanding of issues associated with analysis and theory development. The student experience (if they have any critical awareness) is likely to be frustrating as they realise the limitations of their work, and the project is in danger of becoming a ritual that has to be gone through, for the sake of fulfilling course requirements, rather than a significant learning experience. The stresses of doing research are considerable, even with the best possible support: attempting to mount a study with only limited teaching input and opportunity for debate is likely only to increase this stress.

One argument for these small scale projects is that they do not involve huge resources. This view, however, does not consider the major resource in this type of project – i.e. staff time. There has been a debate in the nursing press about this issue (Barlow 1988) which conjures up images of ward staff being constantly pursued by nurses on courses carrying notepads and tape recorders. This is clearly a potentially harmful situation, where nursing time is spent with researchers, and patient care is disrupted. This approach to teaching research methods is, therefore, questionable – particularly as there is little possibility of any meaningful results being produced by the research.

With these issues in mind, during the planning of the part time BSc (Hons) Nursing Science programme for qualified nurses, the course team decided on tackling research through a group project. The advantages would be that students would have a supportive environment in which to explore research issues, without the problems of having to conduct an independent study. This strategy, it was hoped, would reduce the need for intensive supervision for independent projects, time that would be disproportionate to the emphasis placed on this component within the course. The course is, after all, not a research degree, but a nursing degree, and there are a number of other, equally valuable areas to be covered.

We also made a decision that, as far as possible, the group project would use readily available secondary data, rather than interview, questionnaire, and observation data. We defined secondary data as 'data which had already been collected for purposes other than the research'. This would minimise inconvenience to research subjects, involve less time in data collection, and would raise the same methodological issues as primary data, for example sampling strategies and interpretation of findings.

Since making these decisions, we have run the group empirical project twice, with two different intakes. In the first intake the students collected memos, which were analysed in the context of organisational communication. For the second intake the secondary data source used was off-duty rostas, these were analysed in the context of staff organisation. The group project is extremely time-consuming – it lasts throughout the whole first year of the course, with approximately two hours of weekly teaching for 30 weeks. It is important that students are able to attend most of the sessions otherwise the continuity of the project would be lost. This chapter describes our experiences in setting up and then teaching the students research methods using a group approach to data collection. It highlights the difficulties we encountered and describes some of the ways in which we overcame these difficulties. It also discusses the strengths and limitations of this approach as a method of teaching research and the wider impact that this approach had on the dynamics of the student group.

THE STUDENT GROUP

The students were all qualified nurses who had completed either the London Diploma in Nursing or the CNAA Diploma in Professional Studies in Nursing at some time in the past. They came from a variety of clinical backgrounds including psychiatric nursing, midwifery, community nursing, paediatric nursing as well as general nursing, and were at different stages in their careers. In addition, a number of the students were not clinicians, but were teachers or managers. These factors obviously produced a very heterogenous group, in addition to the usual differences in learning styles and personalities. It also gave rise to a great deal of diversity in their understanding and experience of research methods. It was important, however that at the end of this course component all students achieved a similar level of understanding of research methods.

The course aimed, however, to do more than just enable the students to conduct a small and fairly narrowly defined piece of research. As the above discussion indicates, it aimed to develop the students' understanding of the wide variety of approaches to research which are open to nursing and to enable them to understand the implications of adopting each approach.

The overall objective was to allow students to develop insight into the issues and decisions which arise in a research study, and to equip them with a sound understanding of the decision making process in research. It was hoped that this would enable them to conduct their own study at some time in the future. In addition, it was apparent at diploma level that students either had an over-respectful view of research, in that they tended to accept research findings without criticism, or conversely that they were idealistic, in that the smallest flaw in a study would lead them to reject the findings completely. Hopefully, by taking the students through the process of conducting a project, their understanding would allow them to use research more appropriately in their work.

ORGANISING THE PROJECT

Setting up the research projects involved a considerable amount of behind-the-scenes work by lecturers to determine the feasibility of the research. Having made the decision to use secondary data as far as possible the first stage was to identify a suitable source of secondary data that was easily accessible to all, or most, of the students on the course. In the light of this we opted for memos in the first study and off-duty rosters in the second study. The preliminary stages involved doing a literature search, clearing the project with ethics committees, and conducting a pilot study.

The literature search in both cases yielded very little in the way of substantial research efforts on which to base the group studies. There was a body of organisational theory which had relevance to the first project, but very little empirical research about communication between staff in health care organisations. Similarly there was little research concerning planning off-duty rosters to be found, although there was some literature of an anecdotal nature which looked at different methods of rostering.

This dearth of literature did not present many problems for the group project, in that it clearly indicated an exploratory study rather than a hypothesis testing study. This, we felt, was actually an advantage, in that a descriptive project can be developed up to the level of hypothesis testing, thus offering the students insight into both qualitative and experimental research. If we had been able to identify clearly a hypothesis from the literature, not only would the project be less creative, but it would have been difficult to extend the group discussion from theory testing to theory generation.

A more important problem raised by the literature search was the lack of discussion of the use of secondary data. It would appear that these data are not addressed by many texts, or if they are, it is dealt with in a rather simplistic way. Secondary data are often treated as if they were an unproblematic source of information, with validity and reliability taken for granted, which is clearly inadequate. A more relevant discussion is found in texts dealing with life-history methodology, which draws upon diaries, but this type of data is very different from the data we were using (Reed 1992). At the other end of the scale, some texts look at official statistics, for example census data, and examine the process by which these are collected. These texts are interesting, and some of the issues were relevant to our projects, but again the type of data is very different. It was clear, then, from this literature search, that there would be no easy protocols for the collection and analysis of secondary data, therefore we needed to address issues of secondary data collection as they arose.

A major issue confronting the use of secondary data derives from the fact that it was not written specifically for the research, therefore it is not tailored to the research question(s). This can mean that when it is collected it is de-contextualised or taken out of context. In these circumstances it is important not to make assumptions about the data. For instance the students using the off-duty data had to resist the temptation to comment on staffing levels and skill mix; this would have required the addition of workload indicators which were not available to the group. This highlights the temptation, which students often feel, of generalising beyond the data.

Having looked at the literature, we were then able to develop a research proposal to take to the various different health authorities involved. This was a time consuming process, which involved attending a number of committees, and modifying the proposals in light of their comments. Some health authorities had clear procedures for dealing with research proposals, whereas others did not appear to have any clear mechanisms, and so some students had to negotiate independently with their managers for permission to collect data.

After approval from the health authorities was given, the teaching staff then conducted pilot studies. A small amount of data was collected, and examined to ascertain whether it was capable of generating useful research and analytic issues. The pilot studies also allowed the lecturers to identify postential problems with the project, and to sketch out possible analytic procedures. The possibilities of the data which the lecturers identified served to shape the ensuing group work, not necessarily in a coercive way, as the project remained open to new suggestions from the students, but these ideas did serve to give an overall focus to the projects.

This preliminary work was conducted before the course began, without the participation of the students. In this way it deviates from the ideals of a student generated project, with the consequent feeling of ownership that that would produce. In essence the topic and method of data collection was determined by the lecturers, and indeed the conclusions were anticipated from the pilot work.

Throughout the whole project this issue was one which the lecturers had to confront, the tension between being so over-directive that the exercise became one in which the students unenthusiastically followed our instructions, and learned little in consequence, and being so under-directive that the project drifted into chaos. For instance many of the students became very frustrated with the limitations of secondary data and were eager to collect primary data, as they felt this was the only way the research could progress. However, we felt it was important for the students to exhaust the possiblities of the secondary data before rushing out to collect primary data with little idea as to why or for what purpose. This did create quite a lot of tension within the group that was sometimes difficult to handle.

A balance had to be struck, therefore, between these two options, encouraging students to enter into the debates and decisions, while still retaining some overall sense of the direction of the project. Maintaining this balance was difficult, however, and on occasion involved some rather underhand strategies, such as allowing the students to spend time in debates we anticipated would be fruitless. Not surprisingly there were periods in both projects when the students were extremely hostile to the lecturers, vacillitating between demanding to be told what to do, or demanding that we stopped interfering with their ideas.

For this reason the course was always taught by two lecturers together, who were able to support each other. Using two lecturers in many ways legitimised the teaching process for the students as they recognised that the issues did not derive from the idiosyncrasies of one lecturer but was instead part of a planned teaching programme. It was important, however, that the lecturers were able to win the confidence of the students, as this was essential to maintain their co-operation.

Introducing the research project to the students

When the students began the course component, the lecturers introduced the project. We gave a rationale for the choice of a group project, and outlined some of the potential problems of such an endeavour. We anticipated that with such a diverse group of students that there would be problems of decision making and reaching a consensus, but the debates were the means by which the students would learn.

When introducing the topic of study, we asked the students to imagine that they had been commissioned to do this research by a health authority. The topics we have chosen have not been popular with the students. In fact they were probably the last areas they would have chosen for themselves, but their response did provide a useful basis for a discussion of research autonomy, and the way in which research is often controlled by sponsors and funding bodies. We also had interesting discussions about what is viewed as useful or important research; from these it emerged that everyday taken-for-granted practices are not viewed as interesting or significant enough for research. This discussion by no means generated great enthusiasm for the project, but it did increase acceptance to some degree.

Looking at the literature

For both projects, the initial group work involved the students in looking at the literature. The lecturers had already covered some of it, but we felt that the students also had to conduct a literature search, not only to uncover some that we might have missed, but also that they could develop skills in looking at the work of others, in order to identify theoretical and methodological issues for their research, rather than looking at literature to guide developments in practice.

We organised the literature search by dividing the class into small groups, and assigning to each one a search method. We are fortunate in having an excellent library which provides a number of different methods of finding literature, including a CD ROM, abstracts, indexes, a current awareness file, and computer catalogues. Before going to the library, the class carried out a brain-storming exercise to produce lists of key-words and subject headings which could access the appropriate area of literature.

The literature search was, as we had predicted, very limited. Initially this produced great frustration in the students, but led to a discussion of the appropriate type of research for an area in which so little had been done. This provided an opportunity to compare and contrast the different research paradigms existing in nursing, i.e. the differences between positivism and naturalism, quantitative and qualitative research, and inductive and deductive theory development. We had anticipated that in the first instance the research would be exploratory. During the overview of different research strategies the links between exploratory research and the problem faced by the students were emphasised. This encouraged the students to recognise that this was possibly the most appropriate approach to adopt.

Discussing Issues of methodology

Having established a descriptive/exploratory framework and a topic of study we then asked the students to look at research methods. Again we divided them into groups and sent them to the library, each group looking at a different method, and each with a set of questions to answer. The methods were observation, questionnaires, interviews, and secondary data, and the questions were essentially about the ways in which each research method can be used, what sort of information it accesses, and the implications of using it in a structured or unstructured way. The groups were also asked to think about their method in relation to the research topic.

When the groups fed back there was some degree of allegiance to their allocated method, except for the unfortunate group which had drawn secondary data. This group had a number of problems because of the lack of information available, and their presentation did not convince the rest of the group that this approach was viable. Observation was also rejected by the group as they realised the enormous logistic problems of, for example, observing staff communication, or discussions about off-duty. The most popular methods were interviews and questionnaires, which on first examination seemed appropriate and convenient.

We allowed the students to pursue this course for a while, and then started to ask questions about what these interviews or questionnaires would contain. Given the lack of previous work in these areas, the group could not come up with many ideas, and those that were suggested were examined further for their rationale.

From the lecturers' perspective this was, perhaps, the most difficult part of the course as we had to persuade the students to choose secondary data in order to adhere to the protocols we had negotiated with the various health authorities. We also recognised that if the students opted to do questionnaires or interviews, the time involved in setting this up and collecting the data would exceed the time available on the course and the purpose of the course would be lost.

We adopted a strategy which highlighted the need for further information before an appropriate focus for the research could be identified. At the same time we emphasised the need to be pragmatic and to pursue a strategy that was realistic within the time available. As any experienced researcher will testify, such constraints are not uncommon in research as most, if not all, research proposals have to be tailored to the resources available both in terms of time and scope.

Consequently we debated the difficulties of collecting structured and unstructured data using questionnaires and interviews, before steering the discussion towards secondary data, which had initially been dismissed. The class were asked to identify what types of secondary data were available which related to their project. Both intakes were able to identify a variety of material. They were, however, still unsure about how this material could be used. At this point we introduced the pilot work undertaken by the lecturers in preparation for the course and outlined some of the possibilities. Both intakes still had some misgivings about using secondary data, but accepted it on theoretical and pragmatic grounds. Theoretically, this data could generate a number of issues which could form the content of interviews and questionnaires, if we decided to do this at a later date. Pragmatically, the resources and time required for the other methods were seen as prohibitive, while secondary data was at least fairly easy and non-intrusive to collect.

Sampling

Having identified secondary data as an appropriate form of data, the next consideration in both projects was the organisation of data collection. This led to a discussion of sampling strategies. This was explored with both intakes, we did not feel, however, that we covered this area adequately with the first intake. For the second intake we decided to make the discussion more explicit. We therefore adapted the strategy which had worked with the literature search and the research methods, namely, dividing the class into groups and allocating each a sampling strategy to look at. We chose a variety of different strategies, in order to ensure that the students covered both probability and non-probability sampling. One problem was that whereas probability sampling is discussed fully in texts, non-probability sampling is either dismissed as inadequate, or discussed in such a way that implies that it is clearly inferior. We therefore chose theoretical sampling as our example of non-probability sampling, feeling that this would be discussed seriously in those texts which acknowledged it. The language of these texts was, however, very difficult for the students, and so we had to supplement them with summaries of our own.

At the feedback sessions we introduced the discussion with a summary of concepts such as universe and sampling unit, and asked the students to summarise the strategy they had looked at. We then discussed how we could use each strategy. At one point we developed an elaborate strategy which involved cluster, stratified, and random sampling, all used in conjunction. This would have actually been a possible strategy if resources had allowed, but when we referred back to the discussion of sampling universe, it became clear that we had no way of determining this. Stratification was also a dangerous path to tread, as there were no clear indications of what variables would be relevant to define the strata. When discussing theoretical sampling we also had a number of problems, in that we had no theoretical focus to explore. After much debate, we finally decided on convenience sampling, much to the disappointment of some of the students, who had read that this was methodologically weak. Our counter argument was that it was, but that it was the most realistic option open to us, given the lack of time available to the project. What it meant to us was that we would have to be very careful in what we claimed about our results, ensuring that these claims did not over generalise the findings.

Having decided on convenience sampling, we then discussed the mechanics of collecting data. In both projects students identified a collection point, (e.g. a ward), and decided on the timing and the amount of data to be collected. In the first project it was decided that the student would collect the first ten memos which arrived at the ward, starting on a particular date. In the second project the students collected three weeks of off-duty rosters from each identified ward, the same three weeks in each case to avoid the usual off-duty problems around Christmas and New Year.

Data analysis

After three months debating methods and sampling, the data collection itself only took a few weeks. There had been some problems, for example staff throwing memos away in the first project. This was discussed, and it was decided that the internal post was so haphazard at most hospitals, that the sequence of the memos was not important, and the possibility that the memos had been selectively discarded was remote.

The two projects involved different types of data analysis. The first one involved a coding exercise, which was extremely valuable in demonstrating to students how raw data can be developed into something that has a degree of conceptual coherence. It therefore demonstrated the principles of data analysis. Students were asked to identify the full range of potential categories into which the data could be located. Following this exercise the students were then asked to identify and merge similar categories in order to group or cluster the data. As this point we reminded the students of the purpose of the research as it had originally been set up and suggested that they return to original literature review. This greatly facilitated the process of identifying theoretically meaningful categories.

We did, however, make a mistake in how we then dealt with these coded data. Because we wanted the students to explore statistical methods of analysis, and also develop some skills in information technology, we then entered the codes onto a computer package which then looked for correlations between variables. Theoretically this was bordering on the spurious, in that our research was descriptive rather than correlational, and the correlations identified had little validity. Some students, to their credit, identified this problem, which generated a discussion of 'shot-gun' approaches to research, i.e. throwing everything at the research problem in the hope that something will turn up. Some of the class members were, by this time, such polished pragmatists, that they did not really see this as an issue.

For the second project, the data were qualitatively different, so we first looked at it in terms of normal patterns of off-duty. This was done using descriptive statistics, (e.g. means, frequencies, and ratios), and using a computer package to present these in graph form. This allowed students to appreciate the differences between descriptive and inferential statistics, but the results created less excitement than in the first project. The statistical analysis of off-duty rosters showed only that off-duty was boringly uniform whatever the setting or staff levels, with most staff having two days off together, preceded by a half-day or early shift, and followed by a late shift. Interestingly, those wards where this did not happen, were wards where staff chose their own off-duty, suggesting that these patterns are not necessarily what staff want.

These findings, which were 'just what they knew already', failed to interest the students, so we then began to discuss what efforts and considerations went into producing these rotas. This was more interesting, so the group decided to follow up the secondary data with an interview. This was loosely structured, consisting of a few alternative ways of asking the question 'What do you take into consideration when writing the off-duty' and a few loosely defined prompt questions if respondents ran out of ideas.

At the feedback session we used a version of the nominal group technique to collapse the identified factors under coherent titles. This generated 50 factors which nurses had identified. It was stressed that this did not represent a measure of the importance of these factors, neither did it represent the complete range, it only told us that they are acknowledged by some of the nurses we interviewed. We began to attempt to code these factors, but unfortunately the course was coming to an end, and the assignment was due in, so we decided to leave the data at a stage where the coding was clumsy and problematic. Some students developed the coding further, but others abandoned it and simply reproduced the list in their writing up. This was a lost opportunity, as the data analysis in the second project was weak in this type of qualitative analysis, and experience showed that this was a very useful area to develop further, especially as it is skimmed over in many texts. At this stage, however, the pressures were such that we did not have enough time to do it properly. This indicates that the volume of work that has to be undertaken in any research project is very great. It reinforces our original contention that the use of secondary data is a pragmatic solution to the otherwise overwhelming problem of data collection.

Writing the report

The students' reports in both projects demonstrated a tension between describing the process of learning, and presenting the product (i.e. a coherent piece of research). The format most followed was that of the traditional research paper, with sections on literature, sample, methods, and results. This format did not adequately express the learning that had occurred, and it led to internal inconsistencies. After discussing the limitations of the methodology, it was difficult for students to discuss findings in a way that did not appear either dismissive or naive.

There were also some problems of recall, where students could not remember some of the intense discussions, or had not been there when they had occurred. This problem was identified early on in the first project. In order to help the students we developed a research diary. Each student was issued with their own diary fairly early on in the course and advised to complete this diary at the end of each class. The diary consisted of a range of topic headings such as literature search, research methods sub-divided into observation, interview, questionnaire, secondary data. Similarly under sampling a range of different strategies were listed. The students were strongly advised to make notes under the appropriate headings at the end of the respective class and also to insert any references and notes taken from written texts on that topic. Some students concientiously completed the diary and found it a great help when writing up the project. Others were more lax and therefore lacked the notes necessary to write up the project authentically at the end.

In each case the locus of control over the project moved progressively from the lecturers to the students. It was therefore, fairly easy for the lecturers to identify the appropriate headings and sub-headings during the early stages of the project as at this stage they were exercising considerable control over it. However, from the point of data collection onwards, the students increasingly exercised control over what they did with the data they had collected, how they categorised it and analysed it. This meant that for the latter stages it was difficult to predict in advance appropriate headings. The diary for the latter stages was therefore less structured and contained headings like 'Make short notes on how the data was analysed' or 'Discuss the analytic categories developed and why they were chosen'.

We recognise that as well as the diary we need to develop some guidelines for writing up this project which allows students to demonstrate their learning more explicitly. There are a number of possibilities, such as a workbook in which they must discuss issues not necessarily in relation to their project. An example could be a section in which they are required to discuss the pros and cons of different sampling strategies. This would create other problems, however, in that the coherence of the project would be lost, and the experiences the students had undergone would not be fully acknowledged.

It is probable that there will always be a tension between demonstrating learning about research methods, the aim espoused by the lecturers (who are not looking for, or expecting results), and the completion of a piece of research, the aim identified by most of the students. However, the better students were certainly able to demonstrate both aims in their final project. Such tensions do, in fact, help with the grading of the final project. It is worth noting that at the end of both projects the students demonstrated considerable insight into issues of research, more than we personally have witnessed using any other teaching method. For this reason we feel, that despite the trauma for all concerned, this is a useful approach to teaching research.

EVALUATION

All things considered, the student evaluation of both of these projects was surprisingly positive. The first project was evaluated before the research had finished, and at a time when the students were probably in the lowest depths of despair during the coding exercise. Students were asked to fill in an anonymous questionnaire which asked them to evaluate the group project as a means of teaching research. The students seemed to be split into two distinct groups. Roughly half of the group were very positive, making comments such as 'It's the most interesting thing I've ever done on a course'. While the other half were quite negative, making comments such as 'I'm more confused about research than I ever was'.

A year later, the project was evaluated again, as part of the course evaluation, and the responses were much more positive. There were no negative comments apart from a few students who said that at the time it had been awful but, with hindsight, they felt that it had been valuable and had helped them tackle other course work with greater awareness of research methods. The second project was evaluated as part of the overall course year evaluation, when the projects had been written. The response was extremely positive, with the exception of one student who claimed to have found the work on off-duty rosters boring, and hadn't understood what was going on. Unfortunately, with anonymous questionnaires, there was no way of finding out any more about this student's problems. Some students commented that, initially, they had found the project difficult, or had gone through periods of despair when they felt they would never understand the research, but that this had passed, particularly when they came to write up the project. This suggests that the writing up may be very important in consolidating learning, with some students only making sense of what has happened when they do this.

Overall the students demonstrated a very good grasp of complex methodological issues at the end of the project. From the lecturers' perspective it certainly seemed to be a very successful teaching strategy. It produces students who are not only able to appreciate issues of methodology, but who also possess a pragmatic and realistic view of the constraints under which researchers work. This is an important learning experience which enables the students to accept the limitations of research. This is demonstrated in other aspects of the course where the students no longer search for the 'definitive' piece of research, but instead recognise the need to set research within a theoretical and ideological context.

Considering the anxiety and hostility expressed by the students through-out the project, it is extremely pleasing to find that, at the end of it, they do feel that it has all been worthwhile. One of the main causes of student anxiety appears to be their lack of confidence in the teachers. Especially in the initial stages of the research, when all seems vague and ill-defined, students are prone to blame this on the teacher's incompetence as a researcher. As all they have ever seen of research is the finished and polished product, they find it difficult to accept that all projects go through this initial stage, and they therefore assume that it is because the lecturers do not know what they are doing. Having two people teaching goes some way towards overcoming this problem. The lecturers are able to support each other – which is important when the students are doubting their competence. Moreover, their combined experience in research can be used to reinforce their credibility as lecturers when the students express insecurity.

It is important, however, that the two lecturers have a good working relationship, and discuss the project before and after each session, so that they both know what they are trying to achieve. Without this, the project can be pulled in two directions, and when students realise this their anxiety increases.

In addition to a good rapport, the lecturers also need substantial experi-ence in doing research themselves. This not only gives credibility, but it is invaluable in answering surprise questions, predicting the consequences of the group's decisions, and relating the group work to wider methodological issues. In this type of teaching, you need to be at least one step ahead of the students all the way. Knowing about research from textbooks can get you through some issues, but it does not provide all the answers or anticipate the likely problems. In its formative stages, research is messy and confusing: the students experience both the mess and the confusion. If these aspects are not to overwhelm the course, then it is important that the lecturers feel comfortable with this, know it to be an essential component of research and are not disconcerted by it. Arguably this requires considerable research experience on the part of the lecturers if they are not to be as overwhelmed by the experience as the students.

In this chapter we have described our approach to teaching research methods which involves the students in the experience of data collection. This allows students to develop an insight into the processes of research which will give them a good grounding if they wish to undertake their own research in the future. We recognise, however, that this process is not essential to developing skills in research appreciation (Clarke and Sleep 1991), which can be achieved in other ways. Instead we have presented our experiences in tackling the difficult problem of teaching research methods using the approach outlined above. We think we have clearly demonstrated the resources required both in terms of time and expertise on the part of the lecturers to undertake this approach. We would argue that if a group project is so demanding on the students, even though it is well supported by two lecturers experienced in the field of research, then individual projects probably require an even greater amount of resources and expertise. However, if the expertise is available and the time can be found in the curriculum we would recommend this approach as a satisfying and dynamic method of teaching which produces some excellent results in relation to student learning.

It is apparent that this approach to teaching depends on careful lecturer control and monitoring. This raises the question of whether the exercise is truly androgogical and student-centred. The degree of control the students have over the research project is limited, in fact part of the lecturers' role is to determine what decisions can be safely left to the students and what cannot. The lecturer's role is therefore extremely manipulative, for example when the group are heading towards a disastrous decision, the lecturers need to anticipate this and guide them in another direction. This has usually been done during debates, pointing out the consequences, either theoretical or pragmatic, of different courses of action. In many ways this type of teaching reflects some of the notions about 'reflection-in-action' put forward by Schon (1987). Through these debates, the lecturers articulate their thinking processes and problem solving strategies. These are made explicit to the students and indeed many of the students come to adopt these patterns of thinking about research problems as the course progresses. In this sense the lecturer control is not purely didactic, but instead is designed to facilitate student learning through a process of setting and solving problems.

This issue of control underlies Schon's discussion of the coaching function of the teacher. Setting up a practicum, and coaching students through activities, clearly depends on the teacher's expert knowledge of what is relevant and important to explore in the learning experience. Hence this type of teaching cannot be student controlled to any great extent. Students can make decisions, but the impact of these decisions must be explored with the teacher/coach so that when these issues arise in the 'real world', the student can begin to predict or anticipate outcomes. If we accept that the teacher is there in the practicum by virtue of expertise, and that the students are there by virtue of their inexperience, then it is difficult to see how learning could occur without some degree of control and structure.

Hence the facilitation of reflective practice may not sit easily in a democratic, androgogical, student-centred ethos, and perhaps this is a major issue facing nurse educators at this time. In moving from the 'knowledge as facts' didactic approach to education, which has been recognised as limited, we cannot move to an approach without any degree of structure and control, without compromising the usefulness of the teaching we do. This is because we do not teach for teaching's sake, or because the pursuit of knowledge is an end in itself; in nursing, as in many other applied disciplines, we teach so that students may practice, and whether this practice is research or clinical skills we have to ensure that it is understood, evaluated, and safe.

REFERENCES

Barlow S (1988). Suspect Research Projects. *Nursing Times,* **84** (15), 14.

Clarke, L. and Sleep, J. (1991) Nurse Education Tomorrow Conference. The what and how of teaching research. *Nurse Education Today*, **11** (3), 172–178.

Reed, J. (1992) Secondary data analysis in nursing research. *Journal of Advanced Nursing*, **17** (7), 877–883.

Schön, D.A. (1987) *Educating the Reflective Practitioner*. Jossey-Bass, California.

Section Four
Reflective Exercises

Introduction

The common characteristic of the strategies in this section is that they concentrate on using knowledge, rather than on acquiring it. They assume that students will have gained, through reading, lectures, and experience an overall appreciation of the literature and thought relevant to the debate concerned, and that their need is to learn how to use this knowledge. A central focus of all of these strategies is that they aim to help students to integrate knowledge from a number of different areas, bringing this knowledge together to look at nursing. In our experience, this is often a difficult thing for students to do, they tend to see knowledge as compartmentalised.

The three strategies are very different, however, in the way that they are organised. Critical incident sessions (Chapter Nine) are group discussions, generated by students' accounts of their experiences. This enables the group to share their experiences, and to pool their ideas. The clinical studies assignment (Chapter Ten) is much closer to a formal essay, which is, however, structured to facilitate reflection. This relies very much on individual students and their supervisors discussing the issues together. The use of diaries (Chapter Eleven) is a similar exercise, where students complete a record of their clinical placement in a way which is designed to foster the habit of analysis of experience. All the strategies, however, recognise that this process is often very stressful for students, and so must be carefully and sensitively used. These strategies are not cheap or easy, as they demand the provision of good support for students in terms of teachers' time and library provision. Supervision and discussion can be very intense, and is taxing for teachers, as they attempt to develop the habit of reflection in students.

Facilitating this habit is important. All of these strategies require students to be observant and analytical about their practice. They cannot, in themselves produce reflection-*in*-practice, but they do develop reflection-*on* practice, in other words the retrospective analysis of experience. The hope is that the discipline of completing these exercises will make reflection-*in*-practice more possible. What the strategies in this section offer is the opportunity for students to take time out from the 'hot action' of practice to think about the issues that arise there.

9 Critical incident technique

Ann Smith and Jacqui Russell

USE OF CRITICAL INCIDENTS AS A TEACHING STRATEGY

Flanagan (1954) worked as an aviation psychologist with the United States Air Force during World War II. He developed the critical incident technique as a method of gathering information about effective or ineffective behaviour performed by airline pilots during designated flying missions. Combat veterans were asked to report observations of their own or other's behaviour and derived incidents were collected and categorised. From this wealth of data, analysing the ways in which decisions and choices were made, he was able to uncover important aspects of job performance and types of stressors and conditions which impair or improve performance. He outlined what he considered to be critical requirements of leadership and specific training needs through the identification of effective behaviour and appropriate attitudes. He described the technique as flexible, capable of being modified and adapted to any area of study as seemed appropriate.

There are a variety of ways in which the technique has been used in nursing. Flanagan, together with Gosnell and Fivars used it in order to develop categorisations for assessing student nurse performance (Flanagan et al. 1963). Cormack (1983) described the way in which he used the technique as a means of examining the role of the psychiatric nurse and Rinon (1979) used it to elicit the nurse's psychological role in caring for patients during rehabilitation. Benner (1984) adapted its use to explore the shift from novice to expert practitioner through the identification of competencies of nurses at different levels of skill attainment. A study by Clamp (1984) described how the technique was used in nurse education to increase students' awareness of nurses' attitudes to patients and their level of interpersonal communication skills. Subjects were asked to identify and record positive or negative interactions between nurses and patients or colleagues. The incidents were used as triggers for in-depth discussions concerning the attitudes and behaviour of those involved. Part of Clamp's study focused on the development and use of a manual for nurse teachers to introduce critical incident technique into the curriculum as a teaching strategy. The use of this approach evaluated positively, not least because important areas of concern and interest surfaced that were not covered by traditional content and teaching delivery methods. Subjects felt that the sharing of ideas and experiences was valuable in that this enabled difficult and debatable issues to be brought out into the open. Clamp reported that subjects perceived an overall gain in confidence, self-awareness, sensitivity and in the development of observational skills.

Whilst critical incident technique appears useful as a means of identifying key aspects of nursing, another real value must lie in the ways in which these aspects can be further explored and evaluated against previously held conceptual frameworks, in other words through the process of critical reflection. For our own part, the use of this technique developed over a period of five years. Initially, the main value was seen as lying in the area of interpersonal development and support for students undergoing pre-registration education. The main perceived benefit was the utilisation of a strategy which reflected the philosophy of holistic education, a means of discovering and using incidents considered to be critical to the students, thus entering into their world, its preoccupations and perceptions. We also saw it as a new and exciting teaching method, particularly when pairing it with experiential strategies and as a means of strengthening teacher-student relationships. During the developmental process, we began to realise its potential in other aspects of personal and professional growth and in the exploitation of the dynamic interface between theory and practice (Smith and Russell 1991). The value of the approach became even more obvious with the implementation of a three year undergraduate course, leading to a BSc (Hons) in Nursing Studies and first level registration – a joint venture between the University of Northumbria and Bede College of Nursing. The nature of the course, the amount and kind of theoretical input, the utilisation of various teaching and learning strategies described elsewhere in this book, the readiness and expectations of the student to link theory and practice and the opportunity for more regular and frequent workshops, all contributed to what may be considered to be an effective development.

ORGANISATION OF THE SESSIONS

Guidelines for students have been drawn up based upon those used by Benner (1984: pp. 299–302). The students are asked to record any incident which made a particular impression on them, recording the context in which the incident occurred and what they remember feeling or thinking at the time. These accounts are anonymous, as we felt that students would feel inhibited about exposing themselves publicly, but we have found that many students do sign their names on the accounts, or claim ownership of them in the sessions. The incidents are collected from the students two or three days prior to the workshop and are then categorised by the teachers, looking for common themes or concerns. This process can be exhausting, and we have found it helpful to do this work in small groups rather than alone. This enables the staff to confirm and clarify their ideas about what would be a useful theme for the session, and also what material can be used to discuss the themes. At times, a unique incident is used, when it is considered to provide an opportunity for significant group learning. After identifying themes, and selecting exemplary incidents, staff then formulate the aims of the workshop, and an outline of content and strategies to facilitate exploration. These strategies may include role-plays, games, and group exercises, depending on the focus of the session.

The critical incident sessions are therefore controlled very much by teachers at present. Although the incidents are the students', we make decisions about what is significant and what is not, and how the incidents should be used. This degree of control is probably the only feasible way to handle such personal material, especially with groups who have just begun the course. What we hope to do, however, is to hand over more of the control to students as they become more confident in handling this type of learning.

Each workshop begins with an outline of the general aims of the day and an overview of the content of the critical incidents received. The teachers' identification of the critical themes in the material is presented, with opportunity for students to debate, question, modify, or confirm the teachers' views. This often generates more critical incidents as students discuss experiences that they have not recorded, but which are relevant to the focus of the workshop.

Following this opening discussion, a technique that we have found useful is to look at particular incidents, (described by Clamp (1984) as 'snapshots' of experience), and to use them to reflect upon the relationship of theory and practice. The process is aided through the analysis of responses to various questions:

- What happened in this incident?
- How can it be explained?
- Are there any other conceptual frameworks which might increase our understanding?

The review is achieved through experiential exercises or discussion groups allowing the students to reflect on and analyse theories, feelings, beliefs and values. An important part of this reflection consists of the recognition and assessment of assumptions which are inherent in any particular theoretical stance or individual belief system.

Within this process teachers and students together explore issues drawing on ideas and theories which might offer illumination. In other words all participants are scanning their intellectual horizons for 'best fit' approaches, enabling the development of discrimination and judgement to discern what is considered to be the most appropriate or helpful explanation or approach in a given situation, in a particular context. What is often very clearly indicated is that there is no single 'right' solution to a problem or definitive approach, and that often understanding and analysis is best developed through an eclectic approach, synthesising various theoretical perspectives. Our observations draw us to conclude that students need support and help from peers and teachers in order to come to terms with this both academically and experientially.

Content of the workshops

A wide range of incidents have been collected and categorised to lead discussions on such issues as health beliefs and education, roles and responsibilities, patient 'rights' and advocacy, the concept of caring, aspects of anger, power and control, the unpopular patient, the unpopular student, reacting to and coping with stress, 'successful' nursing, dealing with grief and loss. These subjects may be found elsewhere in the curriculum, but the workshops provide a direct means of discovering and exploring the different bodies of knowledge which nurses draw upon, and evaluating their relevance and limitations in specific situations. Student interest and motivation are high as common experiences are identified and explanations, analysis and guidance become group responsibilities with the teacher acting as facilitator and catalyst.

The workshops have covered a number of different issues, which students have felt to be important to them in their clinical experiences. Not every incident can be included, so part of the teacher's role is to identify themes running through the students' recorded incidents, so that an overall picture of student concerns can be developed. From this process a number of 'exemplary' incidents are identified, which will illustrate issues which are common to the majority of students. This process of selection is made easier by the homogeneity of the critical incidents that the students report. Especially at the early stages of courses, students seem to identify very similar issues.   Some of these issues have been discussed in relation to theoretical literature which may be helpful in understanding incidents, but the emphasis is not on 'finding solutions'. A number of theoretical perspectives are identified, and each applied to the incidents accompanied by a discussion of 'fit', i.e. to what extent the theory is appropriate for practice. Sometimes the conclusion of the discussion may be that a variety of theories may have something each to contribute, or it may be that none of them can adequately explain practice. This process is very similar to that described by Schön, when he discusses the development of 'theories-in-action' by practitioners, and so the workshops provide exemplars for the students, demonstrating how this process might happen.

An example of this type of session was a workshop held after the students' initial placement with community nurses and health visitors, which generated incidents centred mainly around issues concerning health education. Students expressed anxiety, frustration and irritation related to the problematic nature of encouraging health-related behaviour. We were able to cluster the difficulties related to clients beliefs and values, as expressed by the students. These were identified as those gained through patients' previous negative or anxiety-provoking experiences of health care, unrealistic expectations, lack of understanding, motivation, personal preferences, rejection of knowledge or beliefs of health care professionals, economic constraints and perceived emotional or social difficulties.

Examples of excerpts from two of the incidents used in the workshop are given below:

> 'I was in a vision screening clinic with a doctor and a school nurse and a girl (aged about 8 years) came in with her father. During the screening, it seemed evident that she couldn't see anything below the largest top letter on the chart. She had glasses but she wouldn't wear them. Even after the doctor had spent at least 10 minutes explaining the necessity

of wearing the glasses, she and her father did not seem convinced.

I couldn't believe this attitude, especially since the doctor had explained the far-reaching effects that not wearing the glasses could have. The girl was in the remedial class and I think it was not because she was particularly slow but because she couldn't see.'

This incident was explored in groups of four with students role playing father, child, nurse and doctor. The group work acted as a catalyst for general discussion which included topics such as self image in childhood, 'rights' to reject health advice, parental responsibilities, and the issues surrounding attitude formation and change.

Another incident also illustrated a student's exasperation at not being able to change an individual's behaviour through what she saw as reasoned argument.

'. . . The nurse tactfully asked if she was aware of the harmful effects to herself and that her baby could be damaged if she was constantly exposed through passive smoking. N's reply to this was 'I don't believe in any of that rubbish about damaging your health. My husband's father smoked all his life and when the doctor told him he had bad circulation in his legs due to smoking and he must stop, he did but he still died of gangrene in his legs, nothing to do with smoking. Anyway I'm not daft, how can smoke you inhale into your lungs affect your legs? It's just another fad it'll blow over'. The nurse tried to explain the connection but N wasn't having any of it, so we left. Afterwards the nurse said, 'I didn't push those touchy issues too far this time for fear she won't let me in next time and my relationship is damaged permanently' . . . N made me feel completely stuck for words by her speech on smoking. Whilst I felt anxious to make her understand how unreasonable she was being, I felt angry that she thought she knew best and was not going to listen to reason. I would have welcomed the chance to have been able to go back to N and say 'Look at these statistics, you can't deny them'. . .

Teachers enacted the role of N and the district nurse and students were asked to comment on their own feelings about the incident, discuss how it was handled and to think of approaches which might be helpful in future. It seemed apparent that students had not appreciated the knowledge and skills involved in changing attitudes and beliefs. They were disappointed that nurses were able to exert very little influence over some people's health-related behaviour. It seemed that they expected changes to occur through the patient responding to clear direction from the nurse. Although they had been given some teaching on the nature and function of attitudes and of health belief models, they needed help to relate this knowledge to actual experience. A handout produced for students at the end of the session compared their own findings concerning health beliefs with that of Becker (1974). In this way the students were introduced to a wide range of theories which could develop their understanding of the complexities of health education. Rather than present students with a 'magic formula' for changing client's behaviour, we presented them with a variety of perspectives, and discussed their application to practice.

Another issue that has been tackled in a similar way is the students' 'culture shock' when meeting people from different social backgrounds. These experiences prompt students to reassess their own prejudices and biases, as illustrated by the following examples related to lifestyles and family units:

'. . . The incident I have chosen to share was not demanding or difficult but had an impact on my handling of another patient I came into contact with. During one home assessment, I came across a 'well off' mother who came across as being intelligent and coming from a good family. The house was clean and very modern and the children were smart and presentable. However she seemed completely unaware of how to deal with her children. She did nothing to encourage them or help them to develop. My mentor gave suggestions to help both the mother and the children but by the end of the visit it was obvious that the advice had not really registered.

After lunch we went to do another assessment. This time the family lived on a notorious bad housing estate with high unemployment figures. The mother was living with her boyfriend and they were struggling to keep their heads above water. The house was dirty and neglected and the children were poorly clothed. As soon as I entered the house I immediately classed the mother as being a poor mother. Yet during the course of the visit I was amazed to discover how intelligent the mother was and how well she coped with the children and encouraged them.

At the end of the day I compared and contrasted the two visits and I realise that I was wrong to assume that people who come from better backgrounds will be better mothers. I've learned not to judge people because of their background but I look to see what people are themselves.'

This student's account illustrates a process of re-evaluation of beliefs which is often painful. Many students are reluctant to undergo this process, and can view challenges to their beliefs as personal attacks which they react to by becoming more entrenched. The class discussion about this incident therefore had to be very carefully handled. The discussion focused on the use of stereo types as 'rules-of-thumb' for nurses, concluding that sometimes these were useful in establishing general approaches to clients, but that nurses should always be prepared to acknowledge and actively attempt to identify those clients who did not fit such broad descriptions. By asking students to identify potential uses of stereotypes, they were not made to feel that they were being attacked for holding them, and were more able to then discuss the problems of stereotyping patients.

As critical incidents are very personal, teachers need to be sensitive to students' self-esteem, and to respect them as people with a set of values which may be different to the teacher's own. This does not mean that these values cannot be debated or explored, indeed it is arguably a central part of the teacher's role to ensure that this happens, but it needs to be done carefully. The following example illustrates this.

'. . . The incident occurred during a visit with a health visitor. We visited a mother and her 4 month old baby who was failing to thrive. They live in very poor conditions, their flat being dirty and cold. There was no wall paper, just bare plaster on the walls, no carpets on the floor. The kitchen was dirty with food left on plates, bin overflowing and the cooker covered with grease and burnt-on food. The mother was obviously afraid that she was at risk of having her baby taken away from her and was trying her best to improve conditions. Her boyfriend however made her flat open to everyone, who used all their food and left their flat in a mess almost every evening. The mother therefore had no motivation to keep the flat clean and tidy as she knew it was an impossible task and knew that she shouldn't have to clean up after her boyfriend's friends. . . . I felt very annoyed about the situation, feeling the mother should get rid of the boyfriend who made no attempt to do anything and in fact made her life miserable. She was however adamant that she loved him whatever his faults. The situation was totally frustrating. . . . '

This incident was printed out and used as a focus for discussion groups. The students identified what they felt the role of the health visitor should be in this situation and this they saw as primarily protecting the interests of the child through help and guidance to the mother. One group considered that the health visitor should teach the mother assertiveness skills to help her cope with her wayward boyfriend. Students were asked to look at the situation from a different perspective, considering the three individuals as a family unit and to consider the complex nature of interaction and interdependency within the context of a cycle of social deprivation. By asking the students to do this, we gave them the opportunity to move from their 'idealistic' position (which was based very much on what they imagined they would do if they were in this situation), and to look at the issues from the perspective of the family concerned. This drew upon theoretical notions of deprivation and socialisation, but was also an exercise in developing the students' imaginative powers – the ability to see the world through another's eyes.

The critical incident workshops can not only develop students' understanding of clients, but can also enlarge their understanding of their own, and other nurses' behaviour. For example, students often present situations in which they find themselves being 'unfair' to patients, as the following incident shows.

'. . . When we went in I felt really sick because the lady was incontinent and her house conditions were awful. I felt quite guilty because I couldn't go near her although I obviously did. I told the district nurse how I felt and she said that she also felt disgusted but that we couldn't judge people by our own standards and that the lady might have been perfectly happy living the way she did. I find that the care we give is altered by our personal standards and that different visits and their outcomes are determined by our personal values which we sometimes do not hide. The visit we made was not a 'sit down and chat' visit, whereas others were which is obviously unfair and unequal

care.   Nothing we did was right. Every thing was 'totally wrong and
in the wrong order'. I know the lady was in pain but I still felt myself
getting very angry with her . The most demanding thing was to hide my
anger. . . . I think this is an important incident to reflect on since it
seems to me that its very difficult to care for someone whose behaviour
is so difficult.'

This incident was used as material for discussion in conjunction with a
role-playing exercise which used another incident which reflected similar
themes. The discussion focused on the notion of the 'unpopular patient'
and students were reminded of a variety of studies which explore this.
Consideration was given to the ways in which students interpret and
deal with what they saw as inappropriate feelings on their part and
inappropriate behaviour on the part of the patients. Discussion led
on to the socialisation of patients and nurses incorporating aspects of
role theory, principally expectations and role stress. Comparisons were
made with various other theories (e.g. locus of control theory), as ways
of understanding reactions to hospitalisation or incapacity. Again, the
workshop attempted to synthesise theoretical ideas with the students'
experiences, making it clear that the theories were not 'blueprints', but
could perhaps offer a way of understanding a seemingly unalterable pattern
of behaviour, through an analysis of nurses' reactions to patients.

This type of discussion of theoretical literature does seem helpful to
students, allowing them to see how theories can be used critically
and creatively in practice. It does run the risk, however, of reducing
everyday dilemmas to academic debates, with all the connotations that
has of distance, detachment, and abstraction. That is not our intention –
these incidents really happened, and they should not be treated as mere
illustrative case studies of abstract theory. They are incidents in which
students have been involved, in the full sense of the word.

Some issues are not amenable to theoretical discussion; there is little
research or scientific knowledge which can be brought to bear upon them.
If this is the case, then to attempt desperately to 'make a theory fit' is
not only an unproductive exercise, it is also contrary to the principles
of reflective practice. What can be drawn upon, in such instances, are
ideas from philosophy and literature, sources of understanding which
are under-explored in nursing. This can be illustrated by looking at one
workshop conducted early in the undergraduate/RGN course, in which the
critical incidents all focused on one theme – feeling inadequate.

Many of the incidents suggested that the students were feeling a deep
sense of guilt at not being able to live up to their own expectations
of a successful nurse. This appeared to be particularly evident in areas
requiring great skills in sensitivity and tact such as in caring for very
ill or dying patients and their relatives. A student may feel a sense of
inadequacy, feeling that she is not behaving in the most appropriate way
and may compare her own ability with that of a more experienced nurse.
The following incident illustrates this:

'I took the mother to the room where she was going to stay overnight.
She started to cry, I felt that I could not leave her. I closed the door sat

down beside her and held her hand. As I didn't know what to say I just listened, I felt like crying myself. We sat for 40 minutes. She poured her heart out. Later I was praised for the way I coped but I didn't feel as if I had. I felt guilty about talking when others were busy. . . . I kept thinking someone more experienced than me should be dealing with this but I couldn't think of a way of bringing them in. . . . I felt totally drained emotionally.'

Sometimes it seems that students are looking for a recipe for success and feel let down when applying an approach which they feel ought to work, but which does not.

'We had two women in at the same time for mastectomy. One was happy all the time, smiling, telling jokes and in general being the life and soul of the ward. I felt she was hiding her innermost feelings. I sat down and talked to her one afternoon but she assured me that everything was fine. I talked to Sister about this and she said that she had previously had to talk to a lady after the news had been broken that she was going to have her breast removed. She found that the lady broke down crying only after she said 'It's only normal to be upset. Go on, let it all out, have a cry'. The lady said afterwards that this had really helped. After hearing this, I went back to my patient and said something similar but she still wouldn't let it out. I felt absolutely frustrated'.

In the workshop in which the above incident was used we considered evidence to suggest that different people in different circumstances react in different ways and are helped by a variety of approaches. We reviewed what the students considered to be characteristics of a successful nurse, and discussed the problems associated with our professional intolerance of uncertainty (Holden 1990). The key theme of the discussion, however, was the poet Keats' notion of 'negative capability – that is when a man is capable of being in uncertainties, mysteries, doubts, without any irritable reaching after fact and reason.' (Keats, cited by Katz 1986). This idea was enthusiastically debated by the students, who recognised themselves in the definition of a man who does not have negative capability in that he 'cannot feel that he has a personal identity unless he has made up his mind about everything'. (Katz 1986). In this debate both students and staff discussed the pressure they feel to 'look as though they know what they're doing', and the fear of being thought incompetent if indecisiveness is noticed by others. In circumstances like these, the danger is that any action will be preferable to none, uncertainty hidden, and discussion avoided. Such debates have led us to consider again the danger of a mechanistic approach to teaching key nursing skills.

Each workshop is very different and its effectiveness depends on the nature of the investment made by all participants. It requires effort in preparation, and flexibility and creativity as the workshop progresses in order to capitalise on experiences elicited. Discussion of one incident always seems to give rise to numerous other similar ones. For this reason, we have found it best to work in partnership with a colleague and to evaluate our input at the end of each session. This is a process which requires a great deal of trust and mutual support between teachers.

CONCLUSION AND EVALUATION

Evaluation of such a teaching strategy is difficult since its significance cannot be judged in isolation from other teaching and learning approaches in other parts of the courses in which it is used. In attempting to do so, however, it may be considered that overall we need to assess its impact in terms of effectiveness in achieving aims, its benefits in terms of use of resources of people and time, its acceptability in terms of participant satisfaction. Perceived benefits and participant satisfaction can be assessed more easily than overall impact.

Relying on data from formal approaches in end of term/module evaluations and informal approaches such as exercises at the end of workshops, we have found that most students say that they enjoy the workshops and that they help them to look at things from a different standpoint and generate interest in finding out more. They often express appreciation at being given time to share their concerns, acknowledge great benefits from peer support, a sense of relief in knowing that others feel 'the same way' and express feelings of closeness to other participants.

In determining the possible impact of this strategy, critical incident workshops, we have used an illuminative approach, attempting to describe and interpret the effect on participants (both students and teachers). Accurate measurement and prediction of the effects are impossible, but we are beginning to find evidence of students considering, contrasting, questioning and evaluating various theoretical stances, leading us to suggest that in establishing a culture in which this kind of reflection is the norm, the likelihood is that this will have an effect on the ways in which students approach situations outside the classroom. Aspects of a 'hidden curriculum' emerge, values and assumptions implicit within clinical areas, and this appears particularly important for individuals trying to break away from traditional behaviour patterns expected of student nurses.

The strategy is not an easy one since it requires investment by all participants. From the teacher's point of view, we have found it less comfortable than other methods, since it requires an ability to deal with the unexpected and to capitalise on experiences and ideas that emerge as a result of the discussions. As knowledge develops, so does uncertainty and this can pose both an interesting challenge and a sense of unease or disequilibrium. Brookfield (1990) suggests that teachers who develop critical reflection and foster transformative learning are like 'psychological and cultural demolition experts', when they confront students with the notion that a certain way of thinking is only one option among many. He goes on to say that demolition should not be random wilful destruction but requires training and sensitivity. It seems to us that, at variance with the philosophy of holistic education, powerful emotional feelings underpinning a particular cognitive stance are not always taken into account. Our observations lead us to suggest that the teaching strategy we have described is more likely to be able to support students during the potentially stressful learning process than other less interactive approaches.

Using critical incident workshops, we have been able to identify gaps in knowledge, uncertainties and misunderstandings, and what has been rejected or overvalued. This has led to changes of emphasis in the curriculum, providing the basis for further initiatives such as seminars and recommended reading material. There are obvious difficulties associated with the use of retrospective data gained from the recorded incidents, concerning accuracy of descriptions and subconscious editing, but our aim is to enter into the student's world with all its preoccupations and perhaps misunderstandings. We believe that critical incident workshops allow us to gain this access.

We are aware that our concerns that discussions may stay at a superficial level have led us to be directive in formulating the organisation and the principal content of the day. This has led us to set aside some incidents in order to focus on themes we feel to be most significant. Students are given the opportunity to follow up any aspect about which they still feel uncertain or uneasy with a member of the teaching staff at the end of the session, but we are aware that 'rejected incidents' may be seen by their writers as under-valued by teachers. This is a dilemma for us, as we attempt to acknowledge and respect all students' experiences, yet classify some as being 'more important' than others. These 'more important' incidents, on examination, are those which raise issues which appear to be shared by most of the group, and appear from our readings to be fundamental. Our ideas of what is fundamental, however, may not necessarily coincide with the students' ideas, which again raises the question of the degree to which this technique is truly student-centred. We rely at the moment on negotiation with students, hoping that we have created a climate in which students feel free to dispute interpretations with us. This does seem to be happening – at an early stage of development, one of the students was critical of the way in which her incident had been abbreviated and this led us to take a great deal of care that perspectives and ideas are not distorted through the process of editing. Eventually we hope that as the students become acclimatised to the workshops, and their theoretical knowledge increases, they will become more involved, perhaps taking control entirely, in planning the workshops.

More systematic and detailed evaluation is required to determine the value and effectiveness of this strategy. It seems to us to avoid the rigidities and problems associated with a totally subject-centred or objectives-based approach in that it is flexible enough to meet the learning needs of participants by applying and testing knowledge in a relevant and meaningful way. Perhaps most importantly it attempts to create a culture of learning through reflection that perhaps better equips students to cope with challenges and uncertainties within the practice of nursing.

REFERENCES

Becker MH (ed) (1974). The health belief model and personal health behaviour. *Health Education Monographs*, 2, 324–508.

Benner, P. (1984) *From Novice to Expert: Excellence and Power in Clinical Nursing Practice*. Addison Wesley, California.

Brookfield, S. (1990) Using critical incidents to explore learners' assumptions. In Mezirow J and associates. *Fostering Critical Reflection in Adulthood*. Jossey-Bass, California.

Clamp, C. (1984) Learning through incidents: studies in the development and use of critical incidents in the teaching of attitudes in nursing. Unpublished MPhil thesis, Institute of Education, University of London.

Cormack, D. (1983) *Psychiatric Nursing Described*. Churchill Livingstone, Edinburgh.

Flanagan, J. (1954) The critical incident technique. *Psychological Bulletin*, **51**, 327-58.

Flanagan, J., Gosnell, D., Fivars, G. (1963) Evaluating student performance. *American Journal of Nursing*, **63(11)**, 96–99.

Holden, J. (1990) Models, muddles, and medicine. *International Journal of Nursing Studies*. **27(3)**, 223–34.

Katz, J. (1986) *The Silent World of Doctor and Patient*. Free Press, New York.

Rinon, D. (1979) Nurses' perceptions of their psychological role in treating rehabilitation patients: a study employing the Critical Incident technique. *Journal of Advanced Nursing*, **4(4)**, 403–13.

Smith, A, Russell, J. (1991) Using critical learning incidents in nurse education. *Nurse Education Today*, **11**, 284–91.

10 Clinical Studies Assignment

Jan Reed and Susan Procter

INTRODUCTION

There is a long tradition, in all areas of education, of using essays as a means of assessing students' abilities and developing their study skills. There is much to be said for this educational tool, as it can develop a number of key skills in the students. They learn to access, evaluate, and classify literature and other material, they learn to reference correctly, summarise clearly, and use material in the construction of arguments. For many students, the exercise of writing about ideas clarifies them; thinking through an essay structure allows them to understand the debates within an area much more vividly. As a way of facilitating the understanding of a body of knowledge, an essay is an invaluable tool.

Problems arise with the standard essay, however, when the aim is to encourage students to link theory and practice, especially in a student group where the members have different clinical backgrounds, for example the post-registration nursing Diploma and Degree courses. One option is to use an essay title which is generic, in which case there can be problems of relevance and abstraction. Thinking of an issue which is applicable to all of the group is extremely difficult, unless it is couched in extremely abstract terms, for example 'Discuss issues of communication skills in your clinical practice'. This tends to produce essays which are correspondingly abstract and vague. Another option is to use a title which allows for student choice, for example 'Discuss an area taught on the course in relation to your practice'. This type of essay title, while allowing students to focus on areas applicable to them, does not provide them with guidelines for selection and sharpening of focus. It can produce essays in which students have attempted to tackle huge areas of knowledge and apply them wholesale to practice, without being selective, or distinguishing between important and minor issues.

The major problem with both of these types of essay, however, is that they do not give students any guidelines about how to relate theory to practice. They reflect a traditional pattern of teaching, in which lecturers give erudite lectures, which the students then attempt to reproduce in their own work. When the purpose of the essay is to facilitate application of theory to practice, the lecture may be abstract, but the expectation is that the essay will not be – the student has to do something with the theory, something that the lecture cannot accommodate. Often the result is that the student distils some improbable and impractical conclusions from the literature, and then concludes by saying that he or she cannot or does not practice in this way. The literature is usually used as criterion by which the student evaluates practice and, as it often does not meet this criterion, the practice is condemned. While some degree of self-evaluation is useful, the extent to which students often dismiss their practice seems an extremely destructive activity – and one which does not facilitate a critical approach to the application of theory. If the aim of the assignment is to foster reflective practice, where theoretical knowledge is selected, modified, and evaluated in terms of its ability to address problems of practice, then the traditional essay is of little use. The students' natural tendency to reify theory and despise practice needs to be re-directed by setting exercises which encourage them to turn their usual approach on its head.

With these issues in mind, we have developed an assignment which allows students to choose their own topic for discussion, but which provides them with a clear structure and guidelines about what type of content they should address, and how it should be evaluated. This package, the Clinical Studies assignment, has gone through a number of modifications, and is still in the process of development, as we learn from our students and their response to the package.

THE PACKAGE

The first version of the clinical assignment was a workbook which students completed, with spaces in the book for them to fill in. It began by asking students to describe their practice, identifying elements, such as staffing levels and patient numbers. It then asked them to identify and discuss two different issues arising from their practice which interested them. These could either be problematic areas, or areas in which staff had developed or introduced innovations in their practice. It was felt that it was important to encourage students to write about the good things they were doing, rather than just the problematic areas, but interestingly, students did not seem to be able to do this. Even where supervisors knew the students were involved in a number of new developments there was a reluctance to write about these.

The reasons given by students for this focus on the negative were numerous. Some felt embarrassed about 'blowing their own trumpet', some did not feel that what they had done was worthy of inclusion in an academic assignment, and some did not recognise what they had done as being valuable. Others preferred to spend their time attempting to 'solve problems', rather than discuss problems that had been solved. The expectation that the assignment would help them 'solve problems' was one that was usually disappointed. Students either could not find literature that gave them the answers, or the answers were impractical. The frustration that this caused led many students to go through a period in which they were hostile to any research or theory, seeing it as useless for their needs. While this is quite a healthy position to take in many ways, it can be counterproductive as some students tended to reject all literature outright and sink into despair.

There were also a number of other problems in the first version of the clinical studies assignment. The requirement to discuss more than one issue in practice did not enable students to discuss any issue in depth, resulting in superficial discussions. The issues selected were often not related to their descriptions of their practice, as these tended to be very general. Students could not be selective about which aspects of practice they included in their descriptions, and so they would try to cram in as much information as possible. This information was frequently unconnected to the issues they wished to discuss later, leading to a rather chaotic assignment. Students who wished to discuss toilet training, for example, would not include information on the number and location of toilets on the ward, but they would discuss the number of consultants and registrars. It was clear that the students were completing the workbook section by section, but were not able to integrate the sections to produce a coherent piece of work.

There were clearly problems of integration and focus with this assignment, problems which were not helped by the workbook layout. This fragmented students' material, and did not allow them to appreciate the links between the different sections; they could not grasp the overall structure of their work at the outset. There were also a number of practical problems with the workbook format; spaces allowed could not accommodate differences in handwriting, and those who used wordprocessors or typewriters were disadvantaged. Furthermore the workbook format discouraged re-drafting, an essential part of crafting a piece of work, involving trying out different structures and different arguments. The second version therefore moved away from a workbook format to a less rigidly controlled structure, consisting of a set of guidelines. Students could then present their material in whatever way they chose.

THE REVISED PACKAGE

The second version asked students to focus only on one aspect of care, and gave much clearer guidelines on what was required, and the purpose of the assignment. This, it was hoped, would allow students to 'get their teeth into something substantial', and allow them to integrate their descriptions of practice, their literature review, and their conclusions. The emphasis was much more clearly on starting off from a practice viewpoint, and evaluating the literature in terms of its usefulness for practice. It was emphasised that practice is contextualised, rather than abstract, and that this context should not be dismissed.

Section One – Description of practice

The first section asks students to describe their practice, emphasising that this should only include information which is relevant to and justifies the study of the issue that they wish to discuss. This ability to be selective is a difficult one to develop, as students often take so much of their environment for granted, and it is so complex, that they 'can't see the wood for trees'. Starting to disentangle all of the various aspects of the clinical environment, and evaluating their impact on practice, is, however, a useful skill. Attempting to change or develop practice involves this type of analysis; the practitioner needs to understand what affects what, and what is connected to what. This knowledge or understanding is often tacit knowledge, not often articulated or discussed, so this part of the clinical studies assignment represents an attempt to bring this knowledge into view. This demonstrates to the student how much they do know, and how important this knowledge is. It is important not only because it enables them to function effectively, but also because it is a unique and contextualised form of expertise, as valid as that found in the more generalised knowledge of textbooks. It is this knowledge that tells them what is actual and what is possible. Bringing this knowledge into view enables students to evaluate it, modify it and question it, and to distinguish between major and minor issues in ways that may not have been available to them before.

Section Two – Review of the literature

The clinical studies assignment deliberately starts off from the practice perspective before moving on to the literature. This emphasises the importance of clinical work and clinical issues as the criteria by which theory and research should be evaluated. The second section requires the students to give an overview of the literature that they have found, which relates to the issue that they have identified. The guidelines encourage students to be critical of the material they find, and to evaluate it in terms of its nature and content. A summary of types of literature, and the questions which should be asked of each type is given to encourage students to develop the ability to debate the validity of material.

At this point in the assignment, students are asked to evaluate literature on its own terms, suspending issues of relevance temporarily. Although this, in some ways, contradicts the aims of the assignment, it does encourage and enable students to address issues of methodology and epistemology, in other words to examine the various types of knowledge that can inform practice, and their scope and nature. Having evaluated literature on its own terms, they are then more able to discuss its relevance to their own practice; trying to examine validity and relevance at the same time can often result in neither being adequately discussed. Giving the students some space to look at validity and the general consensus or debates in the literature prepares them for the third section of the assignment.

Section Three – Integrating theory with practice

The third section of the assignment is where, hopefully, the ideas and issues the students have discussed are integrated. The implications or recommendations for practice that they have identified from the literature are examined in relation to the particular and unique circumstances in which they practice. These circumstances are the criteria for the evaluation of the literature; in other words, students consider whether or not it is helpful to them. There are many reasons why the literature might not be considered helpful. Firstly, the research findings may be contradictory or inconclusive, providing no clear indications for policy. If this is the case (and it is common) then the student may wish to discuss what might constitute safe practice rather than effective practice, drawing upon basic theoretical principles, or perhaps evaluate different possibilities in terms of their logical rationale. Some students in this situation have debated issues such as accountability in situations of uncertain knowledge, whereas others have attempted to describe a research programme which might resolve some of the contradictions in the literature.

Secondly, the literature might not relate to the clinical area of the student. This does not automatically make the literature irrelevant, but it does mean that direct application is harder to identify. Students with this problem need to assess carefully the similarities and differences between their clinical area, and the research setting. There are often a number of points in common between seemingly diverse clinical areas, and these may be felt significant enough to allow students to relate the literature to their practice. Conversely, significant differences in setting may result in the conclusion that the literature is not relevant, despite some similarities being identified. Often in these circumstances, where direct application is not identified, students discuss how recommendations for practice could be modified. Other students choose to debate the fact that research into a problem has not been done in their area, and discuss the possible reasons for this deficit, whether these be personal or political.

A third common reason for the literature being unhelpful is that it suggests practices which are not feasible in the student's circumstances. Some literature may suggest increases in staff, intensive training, organisational changes, or the provision of expensive facilities. In this situation students often discuss the feasibility of such changes, and may wish to discuss the cost of changes in relation to the benefits. Others relate such potential changes to wider political and professional issues, such as nurse autonomy, control of budgets, and status within health care organisations.

Occasionally the literature does produce clear and feasible suggestions for developing practice (for example, research evaluating different forms of pre-operative skin preparation clearly indicates that shaving incision areas increases the incidence of wound infection). If this is the case, then the student may wish to discuss how this can be done, or develop a plan of action. The literature may confirm practice, in that it supports current ways of working, in which case students may wish to expand upon this to elaborate further on the rationale they have for their nursing care. This exercise is often very useful, in that it again can bring tacit knowledge into view, validating it and debating it.

EVALUATION

The current version of the clinical studies assignment is not without its problems. There are a number of areas which students find difficult to do, and about which they express a great deal of concern. The most common student problem is the first section, in which students are uncomfortable because they have to write without using many references. This perhaps reflects the process of academic socialisation that they have begun, in that they feel that the number of references that they use is a measure of the quality of their work. This is an extremely difficult problem for both staff and students, because in many ways this view has been encouraged by the academic experience. When students begin courses, they often participate in study skills sessions, which stress the importance of supporting arguments with references. This often produces a situation where students feel nervous about writing anything without references, to the extent that they almost use them as punctuation – every full stop is preceded by a reference, no matter how spurious. Supporting arguments is of course important, but many students come to believe that references have an intrinsic value, rather than one dependant on context and content. Overcoming the fear of reference-less text, is difficult, but it does encourage students to use references more appropriately and meaningfully.

A related problem occurs in sections two and three, where students lack the confidence to critique literature. Again this is often due to an over-respectful approach to the printed page, which accords equal merit to an opinionated reader's letter and a closely and carefully argued discussion article. Once students are coached through the process of evaluating literature, and the clinical studies assignment is one vehicle for doing this, they can learn to distinguish between types of material. The clinical studies assignment is supported by research appreciation sessions, but the timing of these sessions is problematic. If done too early in the course, before students have read much research, it can be meaningless, but if done too late students can feel disadvantaged. Our strategy on the DPSN has been to leave the research appreciation sessions to the second year, and concentrate in the first year on a 'common sense' approach to reading research. We see the importance of the first year as encouraging a healthy scepticism to literature before we introduce complex issues such as sampling strategies in the second year. If this attitude is not developed, then the formal sessions can turn into a 'recipe-book' approach to the research critique. It must be said however, that many of our students do not agree with us, and want taught sessions earlier in the course, so we are at the moment attempting to develop an approach which will both encourage initiative and confidence, and provide a framework for reading literature.

A related problem is the relationship between taught sessions and this assignment, and the extent to which taught sessions provide students with exemplars. We commented earlier that the traditional essay mirrors the traditional lecture, which simplifies the student task – all they have to do is reproduce the lecture in their essay. The clinical studies assignment has no programme of lectures as such, and students are expected to draw from the taught component what they feel is relevant to them. This frees students in one sense, in that they can exercise control over their work, but it disadvantages them in another sense, in that they are not explicitly coached through this process, except in tutorials. As the clinical studies assignment often requires students to synthesise literature from a variety of different disciplines, their problems are increased, as each discipline is traditionally taught in isolation from the others. This is desirable, as students can appreciate the focus, concerns and remit of each discipline, but it does not help students to link disciplines or theories to each other, or to their practice. We have attempted to overcome this by organising multi-disciplinary seminars devoted to subjects such as pain or depression, where a number of disciplines have a contribution to make. These have been successful, and enjoyed by students, but they are extremely expensive in terms of staff/student ratios, as they may require as many as four or five specialist staff to attend (for example physiologists, sociologists, and psychologists) as well as nursing staff. In addition they are difficult to co-ordinate and organise. We may have to resort to holding these seminars with only one member of staff present, a nurse lecturer, which will be cheaper in terms of staff costs, but will not provide students with in depth insight into the perspectives discussed, or provide them with such a rich variety of approaches.

The benefits of the clinical studies assignment have been considerable. Students are introduced to the ideas of structuring work, which allows them to focus on content. In our experience asking students to address both content and structure at the same time frequently drives them to despair. For more academically experienced students on the part-time nursing degree, the structure is also useful, as it prevents them from wandering off into the realms of abstraction, a tempting journey for those who are enthusiastically embracing the world of theoretical debates. There is nothing wrong with this development, but it can become a problem if students completely forsake the world of pragmatic and mundane issues – which is, after all, the world in which they practice, and which is all too easily devalued.

Affirming the importance of the clinical world is a central theme of the clinical studies assignment, and this appears to be promoted by asking students to describe and prioritise clinical practice. Developing the skills of selectivity, and giving students freedom to write from their personal perspective, facilitates reflection on practice in a supportive setting. Perhaps most pleasingly, many clinical studies assignments have resulted in practice developments, where students have discussed the ideas developed in the assignment with colleagues at work, and have applied them to practice. Some students have developed their assignment into a discussion paper which they have presented to managers with successful results, suggesting that the assignment can also empower nurses. These outcomes suggest that the assignment can be compared to a form of action research, where local problems are tackled at a local level.

This does not imply that students cannot identify issues at a wider level than their own practice. Appreciating the importance of policy and political issues in determining care is an important development, adding another dimension to reflection. In this sense, students who can see beyond immediate issues are not necessarily moving away from practice issues, they are simply seeing them in a wider context. The danger of discouraging students from tackling such issues, under the pretext of reflective practice, is that students are effectively 'kept in their place' by academics once again. Penalising students who relate their practice to issues affecting all health care at a fundamental level, does not empower or equip them to deal with these issues.

FURTHER DEVELOPMENTS

Although student evaluation has been very positive, with most students feeling that the assignment has been useful to them in their practice, we feel that it can be developed further. One issue that we have not yet tackled is the way in which we might differentiate between the level of skill we require from the different groups we use it with. At present we give similar guidelines to both Diploma and Degree students, the difference being that the Degree students are explicitly encouraged to discuss organisational and policy issues. The problem with this approach is that Diploma students who wish to explore these issues are not encouraged. The question is whether this type of discussion reflects a more advanced level of functioning, and so can only be expected of the degree students, or whether we can expect both groups to tackle these areas, but that we should differentiate between the level of insight we expect the different groups to achieve. Another similar dilemma is the possibility that we might ask the degree group to outline a plan for developing practice, and indicate how they would implement and evaluate this. This would involve thinking the issues through to the clinical area, and might make the assignment of more use to students in their practice. Again, however, we run the risk of failing to develop the potential of the Diploma group by not offering them this opportunity.

The problems involved in using the same assignment at different academic levels are thorny ones. We obviously need to clarify the differences in our expectations of each group, without disadvantaging those Diploma students who arc as able as the Degree group. This chapter provides an illustration of this dilemma which will be discussed more fully in Chapters Twelve and Thirteen. It is probably enough to say here that assignments which seek to promote reflective practice cannot rely on traditional academic criteria for determining expected levels of ability. Whereas many subjects can be thought of in terms of basic and advanced levels, because the subject becomes more complex or more knowledge is required as students progress, it is by no means clear that reflective practice can be thought of in the same way or, indeed, what these different levels of ability might look like.

Appendix to Chapter 10

CLINICAL STUDIES ASSIGNMENT

GUIDELINES

This programme is seen as an integral part of the course. It provides you with an opportunity to explore the links between theoretical issues in nursing, and an aspect of your professional practice. As this is an innovative part of the course, these guidelines have been developed in order to help you to structure and organise the assignment.

Supervision
These guidelines will be supplemented by advice from your personal supervisor in relation to your chosen topic. It is, however, your responsibility to make appointments with your supervisor in order to discuss the development of this assignment. We recommend that you do this.

It is essential that the study addresses a relevant clinical issue and that prior approval of your choice of topic is obtained from the course leader or other nursing lecturer.

Choice of a topic
In this assignment you are expected to identify an aspect of clinical practice that you wish to explore in more depth. This topic may relate to:

- An aspect of clinical practice that is difficult or problematic;
- An account of a recent change in clinical practice;
- A discussion of a recent achievement, innovation or development in practice with which you have been involved;
- An example of excellent practice you have observed or been involved with.

Structuring the assignment
In order to complete this assignment you are expected to organise it into four sections.

Section One – In this section you will identify the aspect of practice you wish to address.

Section Two – In this section you will review relevant literature in relation to your chosen topic.

Section Three – in this section you will synthesise your description of practice with the theoretical perspectives identified in your literature review.

Section Four – References – In this section you should reference all the texts used throughout your assignment.

Word length

The maximum word length for this assignment is 4,500 words.

You are advised to adhere to this word length and to seek advice from your supervisor if you are going to exceed it.

SECTION ONE

MAXIMUM WORD LENGTH 1,500 WORDS

Description of practice
In this section you are asked to clearly identify the aspect of practice you wish to explore in the assignment. This will involve a discussion of the practical and pragmatic aspects of the issue as it arises in clinical practice.

You should indicate why you are interested in this aspect of practice. This could be derived from an increase in your knowledge or understanding about the issue which has led you to question aspects of practice. In this case you must identify the source of knowledge. If it involves literature you have read, then briefly summarise the literature and reference it. If it is derived from some other source e.g. study days, seminars or discussions with colleagues, then briefly describe how this occurred and why it changed your understanding.

Another reason for your choice of topic may be a difficult or unresolved aspect of practice that you wish to explore further. In this case describe this aspect of practice, illustrating your description with examples or case studies.

It is expected that this section will include a description of your clinical environment. This may include:

- The method of organising the delivery of care;
- Typical staffing levels and skill mix;
- Your role in the clinical environment;

- Typical daily routines, procedures, and patterns of nursing care;
- Other factors you feel are important.

The above categories are examples of things you may wish to include in this section. Some description of your clinical environment, case mix, and/or patient/client care is absolutely essential. It is important, however, that you describe only those aspects of your working environment that impinge directly on the issue under consideration. For instance, if you are looking at cross infection in hospital you might need to describe the current arrangements for ward cleaning. A discussion of cross-infection in community care, however, would require some discussion of equipment and services available to clients. It is important therefore that you *select* only those aspects of your working environment that are relevant to the topic under discussion for inclusion in this section.

In completing this study, it is important that you are aware of potential ethical and legal issues that can arise in producing descriptions of practice, particularly in relation to confidentiality. This aspect of the study *must* be discussed with your supervisor. Failure to consult your supervisor or to adhere to the guidance given could result in you failing the assignment.

This section should end with a summary paragraph which clearly states the issue you wish to study in no more than 100 words.

SECTION TWO

MAXIMUM WORD LENGTH 1,500 WORDS

Review of the literature
In this section you are asked to identify and discuss literature that relates to your chosen topic.

You should indicate whether the literature relates explicitly and directly to your chosen topic, e.g. cross infection on an oncology ward, or whether it is more generalised e.g. cross infection in hospital.

Is the literature in agreement i.e. do most of the texts say the same thing? or are there any debates or contradictory findings which are not resolved? If there are you are expected to discuss these debates. You are *NOT* expected to solve them, simply to be aware of them.

You may want to identify the type of literature available, i.e. is a text based on:

1. Opinion, which is not substantiated;
2. A piece of research into the topic;
3. An official report or procedure;
4. A review which considers relevant research and theoretical perspectives.

You may find that the notes given in the study skills sessions held in the first full time block may help you with this aspect of the assignment.

You should end this section with a conclusion which pulls together the main themes to emerge from your literature review and clearly states the points you wish to make.

SECTION THREE

MAXIMUM WORD LENGTH 1,500 WORDS

Integrating theory and practice
In this section you are asked to re-visit the issue you described in section one, and to discuss this issue in relation to the themes identified in the literature in section two.

The following questions can be considered in relation to the issue you are looking at:

- Does the literature have any relevance to the specific issue you have raised?
- Can you draw any conclusions from the literature which indicate possible changes in practice?
- Do you think it would be possible to implement these changes? If so describe how. If not explain why.
- Does your clinical practice highlight deficiencies in the literature, i.e. complexities in practice which are not considered by the literature. What are they?

Degree group only

It may also be helpful to consider the links between theory and practice in relation to levels of analysis, for example:

- What implications, if any, does your analysis have at the level of the individual practitioner/client?
- What implications, if any, does your analysis have at the level of unit/ward organisation, or at the level of interprofessional co-ordination and management of the unit?
- What implications, if any, does your analysis have at the level of the District Health Authority.
- What implications, if any, does your analysis have at the level of National or Governmental policy, or policies produced by professional bodies such as the UKCC or ENB.

This section should end with a conclusion which describes the relationship between the literature and your practice.

SECTION FOUR

References
In this section you should reference all the literature you have cited in your assignment using the Harvard citation system. If you are unsure about this, consult your supervisor or the faculty librarian.

11 Learning diaries

Joanne Bennett and Mike Kingham

'I never travel without my diary. One should always have something sensational to read on the train'.

Oscar Wilde, *The Importance of Being Ernest*.

Whether or not diaries kept by nurses are as sensational as the one recorded by Oscar Wilde is open to question. The practical value of using diaries in nurse education is, however, something that this chapter will explore.

We have all, perhaps, at sometime or another started a diary, and many nurses will be familiar with the keeping of a personal diary. In the information-driven world of today, people are used to carrying filofaxes, memo pads, notebooks and diaries with them, in order to organise and record the information, meetings and events that are part of their busy lives.

The diary is, of course, also associated with the recording of more intimate and personal events, it is the place where people write down their troubles, explore their inner emotional lives and record special occasions and events, to be perused and reflected upon at leisure. Most importantly the diary is usually a private affair, it is not intended for publication, nor is it to be read by family or friends. Perhaps this is why there are so many leather bound, luxury diaries for sale in the gift shops that come complete with a key!

Some diarists, of course become famous and their diaries become part of the public record. Samuel Pepys' diary was kept for nine years, it ran to 1,250,000 words and over 3000 pages. This diary constitutes an historical record of the Stuart Period and gives us important glimpses and insights into aspects of that world: the organisation and conduct of party games; ice-skating in London during the great frost; the mental instability of Isaac Newton; a first night at the theatre watching a Dryden play and importantly for medical historians, a detailed description of the techniques and performance of an early blood transfusion.

Each diarist is the chronicler, in detail, of a particular life-world; Pepys is the chronicler of Stuart England, Anne Frank the adolescent growing up under the Nazi régime, Barbara Castle and Tony Benn the socialists observing and recording the inner world of cabinet government. A walk around any contemporary book shop in Britain should indicate the interest that both publishers and reading public have for diaries, biographies and personal memoirs; these forms of writing consistently feature in the top twenty books at any given time.

Most nurses, then, will be familiar with either the 'famous' diaries alluded to above, or the keeping of personal diaries. However the introduction of systematically kept diaries as part of the nurse education experience is something that needs more detailed consideration. This chapter is about the introduction of learning diaries into an undergraduate nursing programme, a step which on first examination seems straightforward. When we started to discuss how this would be organised and managed, however, it became apparent that there were many complex issues involved, and so this chapter is an account of how we addressed them. We are aware, however, that our approach may not be appropriate for everyone, and so this chapter concludes with a discussion of how diaries may be used in other ways.

DEVELOPING THE DIARY

When we planned the BSc (Hons) Nursing Studies/RGN programme, a full-time undergraduate course also leading to registration, we were aware that a crucial issue facing all nursing courses is the issue of how the link between theory and practice can be established. Although we intended to use critical incident technique on the undergraduate course, we also felt that we needed some additional mechanism for capturing the range of experiences and issues that the students would face. We were guided in our discussion by Boydell's experiential learning model, which sets out the stages of experiential learning, as shown in Fig. 11.1.

We felt that this process of experiential learning would be facilitated if we could find some way of integrating these stages into clinical experience, in other words we needed some assignment or exercise which would take the students through these steps as they were experiencing nursing.

After much discussion, we decided to use a learning diary as part of the programme. This had, we felt, the following methodological advantages over other forms of assignment, for example the traditional essay.

1. The diary allows for the recording of events or issues fairly soon after they have occurred. That is, the emphasis is on getting the student to

---

BOYDELL'S EXPERIMENTAL CYCLE.

(1) EXPERIENCING

(2) SHARING PERCEPTIONS FROM EXPERIENCE

(3) MAKING SENSE OF EXPERIENCE

(4) ABSTRACTING CONCEPTS, GENERALISATIONS AND PRINCIPLES.

(5) APPLYING PRINCIPLES TO EVERYDAY LIFE AND WORK

Fig. 11.1 Adapted from Boydell's (1976) work on Experiential Learning

record, describe, theorise, explain, and puzzle over relatively immediate experiences. The expectation will be that the student will write up his or her thoughts on a nursing experience in the diary, as soon after the experience as possible. This recording of events, issues, and experiences seeks to minimise the problems of recalling events in detail, a week or so, or even longer after the event. Even if events can be crudely recalled, the reliability and validity of the account is likely to be suspect. Can *you* remember what you were doing on Tuesday of last week? We appreciated that students would have to learn to develop the discipline of maintaining their diary on a regular basis, but we felt that this discipline of reflection was a valuable one to learn.

2. The diary form, systematically kept, allows both the student and the teacher to gain insight into and an understanding of processes, sequences, and the time order of events. This kind of understanding or knowledge is crucial to an appreciation of nursing routines, treatment regimens, the path and course of varying illnesses and their effects on patients over time. Understanding care as a process and situating the real life patient in a time perspective is something that diary records can help us to make sense of.

Since the learning diary had to be designed to meet a number of curriculum objectives, i.e. that it should be student centred, process oriented, experientially related and allowing for the development of the reflective practitioner (encapsulating the theory/practice dichotomy) a decision was made to design a form of semi-structured diary. At this stage the possibility of developing an unstructured diary form was considered, one that would provide the student with the opportunity to select experiences meaningful to themselves. However, on balance, the semi-structured diary was selected because it was felt that undergraduate students needed to be offered some kind of direction upon which to base their enquiry.

The areas for reflection and analysis selected for the semi-structured diary were chosen by reference to the key learning outcomes identified for units of study and placement experiences in the curriculum. The semi-structured diary would allow teaching staff to highlight key issues and components of practice that required further detailed consideration by the student. Since the diary was also to be used as a formative assessment process in the course, it was necessary to write guidelines for the students' benefit which explained the role, function and assessment of diaries in the course context. Students may expect to be assessed via essays, assignments, practicals and project work and they may be clear about the form and the nature of the work to be submitted. However, asking students to maintain diaries as part of their work assessment and educational development, and also to share and discuss the personal, experiential insights that this diary material may contain is a very different type of assessment to traditional approaches, and so we felt that we needed to discuss this with them as fully as possible.

The learning diary itself was structured into seven sections, each of which is now described in terms of the instructions given to students, in Fig. 11.2.

SECTION 1: INTRODUCTION

Learning diaries are an essential component of your course and represent part of the formative assessment process which helps ensure that each student achieves the theoretical and practical outcomes of this undergraduate nursing course. The diaries are designed to be intellectually stimulating and facilitate professional growth and development.

Each diary is supplemented by specific learning outcomes for each unit of experience as well as summative evaluations and continuous assessment of practice. You will be provided with two diaries, one of which should be regarded as a working resource and the other a final account of your learning during each unit of experience, this will be discussed with the course supervisors and mentors. The final completed diary will be available to your supervisors and if necessary the Examination Board and it is therefore compulsory that it is completed before the end of the unit of experience.

The diaries will thus provide a portfolio of learning experience illustrating academic and professional development throughout the course and must be retained.

It is envisaged that you will find that the completion of these diaries, and the subsequent discussion engendered, helpful in promoting patient care and sustained professional growth and development.

SECTION 2: A LEARNING DIARY, PURPOSE AND RATIONALE.

Learning diaries provide a record of information, experiences and situations encountered during clinical and community placements. Recognising the importance of personal experience as a starting point for enquiry and reflection, it is essential that this is more than a straight forward account of what has occurred. You should draw upon theoretical sources, your own professional experience and experience of colleagues, mentors and teachers, in an attempt to understand the complex issues involved in professional practice. You should therefore be prepared to illustrate your discussion with references, sources, initial debate and considered review.

The diary can reflect both personal and professional issues which you have found stimulating, challenging, troublesome or puzzling as well as a record of learning and professional development. This will help in a number of ways:

- It will record personal learning experiences which will be reflected upon and transformed into useable knowledge;
- It will help to identify areas requiring clarification and further research;
- It will enable you to develop observation and information gathering skills;
- It will help you to unmask taken-for-granted assumptions regarding health care;
- It will give direction for discussion and analysis during review and reflection sessions;
- It will act as a resource handbook helping direct future studies and reflections upon practice;
- It will provide a focus for discussion with your mentor;
- It will help you, your mentors and teachers to systematically evaluate experiences.

It is vital that you become aware of issues about confidentiality and be selective about what you write and how you present it. This will be discussed both in class and by your mentor. Avoid using names, addresses etc to safeguard the interests of patients/clients.

SECTION 3: OVERVIEW OF CLINICAL OR COMMUNITY ENVIRONMENT
In this section you are asked to consider some of the following aspects of your current clinical or community experience:

- Philosophy of care;
- Environmental influences on care;
- Organisation of care;
- Patterns of care;
- Multidisciplinary aspects of care;
- A typical days experience;
- Achievement of specific learning outcomes.

(Note: Blank diary pages are now left for the student to write up and reflect upon one or some of the themes identified above)

SECTION 4: CARE IN ACTION
In this section you are asked to comment upon specific instances of care you have observed with reference to the following:

- Patient needs, physiological, psychological, social, spiritual and cultural;
- Models of care;
- Nursing activities and their rationale;
- Communication skills;
- Health promotion;
- Involvement of patient, family and/or significant others.

(Again, blank diary pages are left for the student to write up and reflect upon one or some of the themes identified above).

SECTION 5: ANALYSIS OF YOUR CARE
In this section you are asked to consider the care that you gave or helped give to a patient or group of patients. This should include the following:

- Description of care;
- Rationale for care;
- Research underpinning care;
- Personal reflection on quality and delivery of care;
- Strategies for improving care.

(Again, blank diary pages are left for the student to fill in)

SECTION 6: BIBLIOGRAPHY
In this section you should list in the approved way, all the academic reference sources used in this diary. Subsequently you should state all other reference sources and agencies which have been of value in completing the diary.

SECTION 7: ADDITIONAL NOTES
This section allows a space for students to record any miscellaneous thoughts and ideas that they have which may not have been captured in any of the other sections.

Fig. 11.2 The learning diary

Each student was given two copies of the semi-structured diary, one to be regarded as a 'rough draft' working resource, the other to act as a final account of recorded learning and experiences. Due to the unique nature of this approach to learning a second diary was considered essential as the first one allowed students the opportunity to experiment with diary entries, and to identify those aspects of learning/experience that they wished to record formally in the final version that they would present for assessment.

The diary structure therefore allows students in the first instance to recall, identify and describe personal nursing experiences related to their placements. However the diary structure and guidelines make it clear that in order for the experiences to become meaningful, it is necessary for the student to reflect upon and interpret the experience. It is clearly stated in the diary that students are required to provide more than a straightforward account of what has occurred. They are encouraged to relate the experience and then attempt to interpret the experience by drawing upon appropriate knowledge (e.g. nursing theory and practice, research, concepts of health, biological sciences, sociology, psychology, etc.) It was thought that analysis of diary contents should reveal the integration of theory and practice through the student interpreting clinical practice by way of reference to appropriate theory and vice versa. This process corresponds very closely to the experiential cycles described by Boydell (1976).

IMPLEMENTING AND EVALUATING THE LEARNING DIARY

The diary was piloted with the 28 students joining the first year of the BSc (Hons) Nursing Studies/RGN course, between October 1990 and March 1991. Prior to implementing the diary, the nature, purpose and rationale of the diary was explored, firstly with members of the course team and mentors and then formally with the students. This later session was structured to provide students with the opportunity to discuss any concerns or pose any questions they had in relation to the use of the diary. The diary keeping was monitored by supervisors throughout the pilot period and, following completion of the diaries in March, students were encouraged:

1. To identify the strengths of keeping their diaries;
2. To identify the limitations of keeping their diaries;
3. To define future learning goals.

Staff comments on the diaries were then compared with the students' own responses to their diaries. Of crucial importance here was an evaluation of the students' perception of the value and limitations of the diary as a teaching/learning/assessment tool.

Staff evaluation

Most staff involved in evaluating the diaries were impressed by the insight and analysis developed by many of the students. The standard of work ranged from very bald descriptive accounts of care, with little comment or evaluation, to well balanced and penetrating critiques of care. These critiques were not simplistic or idealistic, criticising practitioners for failure to work by the book, but incorporated a rational analysis of why the nurses worked this way, and of the circumstances under which they worked.

One student, for example, when discussing a client that she had visited with a district nurse, provided a very clear discussion of the physiological aspects of his health deficit, but then went on to use aspects of sociology to discuss the care given. In this part of her discussion, she highlighted the central problem facing the nurse she had worked with, which was the conflict between promoting independence and giving care. She identified the difficulties in deciding when 'doing for' the patient became detrimental to his independence.

Another student discussed primary nursing in her diary. She analysed the way that the nurses actually worked on her placement ward, and concluded that they did not really use primary nursing as they had claimed; after lunchtime the staff tended to work as one large team in order to cover breaks and staff having time off. She did not, however, discuss this in a judgemental way, but pointed out, very sensibly, that the way that staff shifts were organised left the nurses with very little choice.

These two examples indicate a level of analysis and reflection which is impressive for first-year students. They had avoided the traps of either being overawed by practice, or of being over-critical of nurses. Their comments showed balance and insight, and they drew upon a wide range of knowledge and perspectives.

The feedback from the supervisors looking at the diaries did, however, raise one issue – that of assessment. The diaries were not formally assessed, and were given no mark, a policy which had been decided on in order to encourage innovation and freedom of expression in the students. Some staff, however, found it difficult to look at the diary material from any other perspective than the traditional academic concern with structure, referencing and style. Although we felt that we could recognise 'good' and 'bad' diaries, we felt that the criteria we used needed further discussion and examination. We are working on this at the moment, and have decided to bring supervisors together to discuss the learning diaries when they are submitted, but this does raise a very important issue which is discussed in greater depth in Chapter Twelve. If we are to encourage reflective practice in students, then we must be very clear about what we mean by this, and how we can recognise it. One way in which we might organise our feedback is to use Boydell's 1976 model to evaluate the extent to which the student has progressed through the experiential cycle.

Student Evaluation

Using nominal group technique for evaluation purposes (Delbecq 1975), a sample of 22 of the students attended a structured evaluation session on the diaries. At this session two questions were posed:

1. How do you feel you have benefitted from the diary?
2. What difficulties did you encounter when using the diary?

Each student was requested to consider the questions privately and write down their responses. The set of 44 answers from the group were evaluated both quantitatively in terms of the frequency and ranking of particular types of response and qualitatively in terms of the meaning of the responses. A number of themes were identified using the nominal group technique. They are summarised, in the students' own words, as follows:

> The diary made you work harder to develop theory.

> The diary was a useful way to analyse the care given and think critically about the reasons for that care.

> The diary gave you a permanent record of experience to reflect upon; The diary forced me to reflect on experience.

> The diary helped develop my ability and confidence to look at health care critically.

> In documenting my experience, it won't be as easily forgotten; Helped bring different kinds of experiences into some kind of logical order; I feel that the main benefit from the learning diary was the encouragement that the layout and structure gave to the recording of my experiences.

> Made you put theory and practice together and look for a reason behind the care given – Made you think in more dcpth and identify areas and issues which would require more detailed study; It made you look at research connected with particular experiences.

> Gave us an excuse to ask lots of questions of people we were in contact with.

> The learning diary gave my mentor and I a basic framework on which to base our debates and discussions.

> Brought out small incidents which took place during the placement which would otherwise have been forgotten.

The above quotations are of course the positive ones, yet they do reflect some of the benefits gained by using diaries, when seen from the students' viewpoint. They also indicate that some of the learning goals and outcomes desired by the curriculum planning team have been internalised, at an early stage in the students' thinking and vocabulary. The concepts contained in the quotations above, namely, research, analysis, questioning, reflection, identifying, documenting, ordering, emotions, incidents, debates are the very stuff that goes into the making of a 'reflective practitioner'.

On the other hand, problems of using the diaries in their current form were also identified. Students had the following points to make.

> I didn't quite understanding what I was expected to write; also there were difficulties with writing experiences up; there were problems

in balancing the description of an experience and the amount of research/theory reflection on it.

The difficulties were that often it was hard to apply an experience to the heading in the diary.

Some of the headings in the diary were hard to interpret.

The students' perceptions of the problems of using the diary in its current form are important. The comments that are given above suggest that some students found it difficult to 'fit' their experience to the diary structure. We can be responsive to these comments, as the students themselves can suggest ways of modifying the diary, improving its structure, making it more appropriate to their experiential needs. In this sense the students themselves begin to be aware of different types of diary and therefore join into a debate with their teachers about alternative forms of diary keeping. Some students seem to be voicing a concern about 'correct language', as the following comment illustrates:

My difficulties came in expressing myself in what would be considered a professional manner . . . and finding a way to express myself that also allowed me to express my feelings . . . and finding the right words to describe any of the experiences that I had had . . . overall I feel I may have been incoherent.

This concern about 'professional manner' suggests that some students may be uncomfortable with writing about their experiences, or find that this type of writing looks 'non-academic'. This raises two issues, firstly that the course team does not have a right to demand self-disclosure from students, and those students who do not wish to do this should be made aware that their decision will be respected. Secondly, those students who would like to record their feelings should not feel inhibited about using non-professional language as they would in a traditional essay. Expressing feelings in academic language is a high-level skill (one that some would say serves only to disguise and intellectualise the emotions), and all we would ask is that those feelings that students choose to express are conveyed clearly and intelligibly. The learning diary that we used was not focused on emotional elements, but for those who wished to record or share these aspects of their experience, we suggested that they keep a separate diary.

The identification of types of problems experienced by students in writing up their diaries has led the course staff to modify the diaries with respect to structure, clarification of some of the headings, guidelines for a more flexible interpretation of the diary entries by students themselves and, of course, a more informed guidance support system from teachers. As we indicated at the beginning of this chapter, since the use of diaries is in essence about recording and understanding processes, teachers and students are involved in constant interactive and feedback with each other over both the diary form and the diary content. The lesson here is that to use diaries effectively in the curriculum is to commit members of the course team to a complex but rewarding organisational challenge which will build and change as the course progresses.

The results of the nominal group evaluation technique were positive and encouraging. They suggested that a number of the original aims for the diaries had been achieved. More importantly, they confirm the importance the students placed upon the diary as a method for integrating theory with practice, as a tool to encourage critical reflection upon care, as well as a valuable method of encouraging self-assessment.

Preliminary analysis of the detailed content of the student diaries by course teachers supports the view that the diary did indeed function to create a bridge between theory and practice. They also appear to have introduced the students to the process of reflection-on-practice. Terms like 'when I thought about it later . . .', or 'I realise now . . .' are frequent. The students do not necessarily draw upon orthodox theory to explain events, but they do show evidence of thinking through an issue.

OTHER POSSIBILITIES OF LEARNING DIARIES

The way that we have used learning diaries is, of course, only one of the many possible ways that they can be developed. Others may wish to use them differently, and this difference will largely be in the degree of structure that teachers wish to impose on the content and organisation of the diary. We have described this 'Diary Continuum' in Fig.11.3.

The unstructured diary form comes closest to the keeping of a personal diary, the individual decides what they want to write, how much they want to write and when they want to write. The semi-structured form is where the nurse educator sets some general guidelines and identifies key themes or categories that the student should focus on and write about. This is the type of diary which we have used. The structured form is where very specific requests for information/data are identified by the teacher. This form of diary might be thought similar to filling in a log, where the respondent records specific events, or frequencies of activities as directed by the teacher. The structure can relate to a number of dimensions of the diary, those that we have identified are the locus of control, the nature of the data or information recorded, and the time and context of recording.

The locus of control

This is an obvious point to make, but as we move across the continuum the locus of control shifts. At one end of the continuum, students are left entirely free to decide what they want to write. Their creativity, freedom to respond to and record anything observed or felt is unrestricted. They have complete autonomy. At the other end of the continuum, what is to be recorded and how it is to be recorded are tightly and strictly specified.

The nature of the data/information recorded

When individuals maintain a diary for their own pleasure or instruction, what they record and the way in which it is recorded is a highly personal matter. If a diary is unstructured then it is likely that it will contain material, for example names and settings, which poses an ethical dilemma to the teacher who wishes to evaluate the diary. If the student has interpreted the term diary in the 'lay sense' i.e. that it is for the private outpourings of an anguished heart, then what it contains is not for the eyes of others. Even if the student is aware from the outset that the diary will be read by others, this does not necessarily mean that the material would always be written with this firmly in mind. If the diary is to be incorporated into the learning evaluation of the student, then the teacher may be faced with a mass of incoherent emotions that cannot and should not be treated in an academic manner. The material is obviously crucial to the student, but the teacher needs to think very carefully about how it can be used. This point is discussed more fully in Chapter Twelve.

It is likely that the material that the student records in an unstructured diary will be of a qualitative nature; reflections, observations, and memories. They may from time to time record quantitative information – for example the numbers of patients or staff, or the frequency of doctors' rounds. If diaries are to be used by a group of students in the context of nurse education, the teacher needs to consider how this mass of qualitative observations and recordings can be used, interpreted and evaluated. Perhaps sessions will be structured into the course, so that students can read excerpts from their diaries and share their problems and observations. Alternatively the teacher may make the diaries and discussion of them part of a structured seminar system or use them as a basis for critical incident workshops (see Chapter Nine). Problems and observations identified by students in their diaries may be the starting point for essay work or assignments, the teacher helping to identify and make explicit some of the issues that the diary brings to light.

However the teacher may so structure the form of the diary that students are directed towards certain themes, issues and topics in advance of their experience of them, and in addition give guidelines on the ways in which information is to be recorded. The identification of a clear form of recording will enable the teacher to evaluate and assess the diary entries

UNSTRUCTURED DIARY	SEMI-STRUCTURED DIARY	STRUCTURED DIARY
STUDENT CENTRED	STUDENT/TEACHER NEGOTIATED	TEACHER CENTERED
QUALITATIVE ORIENTATION	QUALITATIVE OR QUANTITATIVE	QUANTITATIVE ORIENTATION
TIME AND CONTEXT FOR DIARY RECORDING LEFT OPEN TO STUDENT	TIME AND CONTEXT FOR DIARY RECORDING BROADLY DEFINED BY TEACHER	TIME AND CONTEXT FOR DIARY RECORDING SPECIFICALLY DEFINED BY TEACHER

Fig. 11.3   The diary continuum

systematically when completed.

For example, a group of students all having their first experience of a ward situation might be asked to make a list of nursing behaviours/routines that they observed on the ward. Having made the list they might be asked to rank and rate the behaviours in terms of their perception of the relative importance of the routines/behaviours. Any personal commentary on their observations may also be included. The point about this example is that the teacher can systematically retrieve from the sample of student diaries, lists, rankings, ratings and observations. These data can be organised and displayed in such a way that group debate, analysis, and assessment of the common experience can be undertaken.

At the most structured level the diary might take the form of a log whereby students are directed to record incidents quantitatively, for example making frequency counts of events, record a sequences of nursing behaviour, or measure the time allocated to specific tasks. This information can then be systematically analysed for educational and learning purposes.

The point being made here is that the teacher should think in advance not only about the type of data/information being recorded but the ways in which these data need to be retrieved, used or analysed in the context of the course.

The time and context of the diary recording

Another central decision that needs to be made clear to the student at the outset, is the amount of time to be allocated to diary recording. With unstructured diaries the student may be directed to record continuously throughout the course and to make entries when they feel that it is appropriate. The teacher may, however, wish to set up a discontinuous form of recording, specifying the settings, the dates and the times when diaries are to be used. In this way the teacher may give more weighting to some elements of experience than others. It might be more productive to direct the students to make diary entries intensively for a day, a week or even a fortnight, in a given setting and for a specific purpose than to have them maintaining 'general' diaries all of the time.

CONCLUSION

We feel that the learning diary that we have developed has facilitated a degree of reflective practice in our students which is commensurate with their limited nursing experience. It has provided a vehicle for students to record experiences and reflect on them, coached by their personal supervisor. In addition it has allowed them to identify, assess and plan their own learning, by providing them with a way of recording important issues as they arise, which they can then explore. Although the overall structure has been determined by the course team, the diary is very much under the student's control. This is in keeping with general trends in education where the locus of control is moving from the teacher to the student. One would expect this to have a direct effect upon the teaching/learning strategy and subsequent assessment techniques adopted. However, as Jolley (1989) suggests, students are rarely given the opportunity to evaluate their own learning. The use of a learning diary as a student-centered approach to learning and assessment may be one solution to this problem, as well as providing a suitable means for fulfilling the aims outlined at the beginning of this section.

We are continuing to adapt the diaries as our experience increases. Moreover, as the students' experience also increases in using diaries we would hope that they will be able to decide upon the structure themselves, either individually or in a group. The structure we felt necessary at the beginning of the course may well prove restrictive or irrelevant towards the end of the course, and it would be an exercise in reflection to encourage the students to adapt it.

REFERENCES

Boydell, T. (1976) *Experiential Learning.* (Manchester Monograph 5). Department of Adult Education, University of Manchester.

Delbecq, A.L. (1975) *Group Techniques for Programme Planning.* Scott, Foreman and Co., Glenview.

Jolley, M. (1989) The weight of tradition: an historical examination of early educational and curriculum development. In Allan, P. Jolley, M. (eds.) *The Curriculum in Nurse Education. Croom Helm, London.*

Section Five
Assessing Reflective Practice

Introduction

This is the final section of the book. It contains three chapters which address the very important issue of assessment. Assessment is important because it deals with outcomes. Whether the curriculum is product or process based, there is still a need to evaluate the learning of students, not only for them, so that they can have some measure of achievement, but for teachers, so that they can evaluate the strengths and weaknesses of the course. It follows then, that if learning is directed towards an assessment, then this should be in keeping with the style of the programme; it is confusing for all if a course is taught one way and assessed in another.

Assessing reflection is, however, much more complicated than assessing traditional work. The orthodox academic approach, in which written material is assessed according to traditional academic criteria, provides clear guidelines for students and teachers, but may not allow reflective practice to be clearly identified or developed as it will not always fit academic conventions. An additional problem with the academic model is that it ignores the affective part of learning, and so an alternative strategy is developing which attempts to accommodate this. This strategy, which we have termed 'self-reflection', attempts to capture the emotional impact of learning, but in so doing raises a number of additional problems. These are essentially ethical problems about how such assessment material should be handled by teachers, and problems about the way in which such learning should be communicated. Without clear structures, this type of assessment runs the risk of becoming chaotic, and without clear criteria for evaluating such material, learning becomes difficult to identify.

Chapter Thirteen is a continuation of this debate, focusing mainly on the problems of assessing reflective practice. Traditional approaches are described, and their adequacy for identifying reflective practice is debated. This chapter argues that a different approach to practice assessment is needed, and outlines what this might be. This chapter concludes by arguing that, in order to develop an understanding of how we can assess reflective practice, we need to think carefully about the way we conduct assessment, and the way this is viewed by the person being assessed. Changing this, however, may require changing other aspects of education and practice.

This section concludes with Chapter Fourteen, which extends the debate about assessment into the recommendations and debates about post-registration education, which is currently the area of nurse education receiving the most attention from professional bodies and in the nursing press. Developments in this area are crucial for the future of the profession for, having recognised the need to develop pre-registration education, this must be consolidated by developing post-registration education. The issues are complex ones, however, as they involve marrying notions of professional expertise with notions of academic progression. Chapter Fourteen gives an overview of these issues and debates, and examines the principles underlying them.

12 Assessment of relection

Susan Procter and Jan Reed

INTRODUCTION

Assessment is an extremely important issue in education. It is tempting to focus great efforts on developing programmes and approaches to teaching, but to leave the question of assessment to 'sort itself out'. The hope may be that an innovatory programme can be assessed by traditional methods, but if the programme has been developed to facilitate reflective practice, then this is a vain hope. Not only will students have problems in fitting their learning to the conventions of the traditional assessment, but their teachers will have lost an opportunity for reflection themselves. This reflection is about the nature of reflective practice, and how it can be recognised, communicated, and demonstrated.

This chapter highlights the some of the issues associated with assessing reflective practice. It begins with a brief discussion of traditional approaches to assessment in higher education and considers how these might have to be adapted for assignments which aim to assess reflective practice. It identifies two forms of reflective practice assignments; those that equate reflective learning with self-reflection and therefore use self-reflection as a proxy for reflective practice, and those that seek to develop reflection as an intellectual activity.

Each of these approaches has its limitations or deficits. In addition, they can also be counterproductive (or, indeed, destructive) to the development of reflective practice. This is because the act of assessing a student alters the student's way of thinking. An assessment gives the student criteria by which to judge him or herself in future, and indicators of how he or she should develop. If the criteria used to assess the student do not recognise the complexity of reflection and the pitfalls in developing assessment strategies, then the student will also find difficulty in doing so.

This chapter explores these points in some depth, as it appears important to us to spend some time in a close examination of current practice before we can suggest possible developments. The clearest message of this exploration is that what is needed is an integrated form of assessment, if reflective practice is to become a real goal of nurse education, rather than a catch-phrase bandied about at curriculum planning meetings and similar events. An integrated assessment is, however, less simple than it sounds, and so the debate started here is continued into Chapter Thirteen, where the form of such an integrated assessment is explored further, and linked to current ideas in nurse education about the recognition of expertise.

ASSESSMENT OF KNOWLEDGE

The assessment of knowledge is a tradition well established in higher education. The purpose of higher education has been viewed as passing on to students a discrete body of knowledge within a well defined and generally recognisable subject discipline. Such an approach is inherently teacher-centred as both the parameters of the subject and the content are determined by the lecturer and are only exceptionally challenged by the student.

Under this system students can be failed for two reasons:

- The knowledge imparted on the course is incomprehensible to the student and does not explain anything meaningful; therefore the student's reiteration of the knowledge in an assignment is equally unintelligible.

- The student chooses to discuss knowledge that he or she finds relevant but which falls outside the lecturer's conception of relevant knowledge.

In either case the student is failed in order to maintain the integrity of the subject as a shared set of meanings and concepts. To be awarded a pass in the subject the student must demonstrate that they comprehend this body of knowledge at least to a minimum pre-determined level. For a variety, indeed for most disciplines, such an approach is clearly essential. A tremendous amount of time would be wasted if each set of students had to re-define the subject each time they encountered it. Moreover, communication depends on a shared set of assumptions or meanings. It is important for knowledge development that students learn these, otherwise their ability to communicate meaningfully with other students taking a similar course is lost, as each would have developed their own set of definitions and they would not be shared. There would,therefore, be no common ground between students and teachers.

Despite the high degree of consensus surrounding the level or grading of work in higher education the marking criteria used to classify degrees remains vague. Fig. 12.1 provides an outline of the criteria typically used to assess undergraduate work. As can be seen it reflects increasing levels of abstraction in relation to a topic, but gives very few guidelines as to content.

Within the parameters of the subject the absence of explicit marking criteria in relation to content does give the student considerable freedom to explore material from a range of perspectives. Accuracy of the content is implicit in the way marks are awarded and is presupposed in the student's ability to analyse material. Within this system lecturers can operate tight controls on the reading and content of the courses through lectures, seminars and prescribed reading lists. Alternatively a more student-centred approach can be adopted in which lecturers operate less control over the content of the learning material and students can be encouraged to read widely and be innovative in how they assimilate and use the material they have found. In either case, however, the lecturer remains responsible for identifying both the overall content and parameters of the discipline.

The philosophy of technical rationality which governs much of higher education tends to regard problems to do with the application of knowledge in everyday situations, as something that lies outside the domain of the institution. Application consists of what students do with the knowledge after they have acquired it and this is viewed as entirely their own concern. The function of the institution is to pass on knowledge, but not to stipulate how people should use the knowledge they have acquired. This makes the task of the institution relatively simple and assessment fairly straightforward. As described above answers are either right or wrong according to the logic of the discipline which is controlled by the lecturers.

Within this framework assessment is concerned with the student's mastery of the knowledge judged according to criteria that reflect the concerns of higher education and not practice. This reduces the extent to which higher education can involve itself in solving practice problems. The curriculum can be determined by material that interests those in higher education and the relevance to practice is not questioned as higher education makes no claims to solve practice issues. Hermetically sealed within its own definition of appropriate material, higher education never needs to test out the relevance of the knowledge it teaches or take any responsibility for the consequences for students of its choice of content. Students either enter the sealed chamber in order to partake of higher education or remain forever uneducated on the outside.

The introduction of concepts like reflective practice in professional education, however, breaks the seal. Teaching for reflective practice means addressing, in the curriculum, issues of relevance to practitioners daily

Grade	mark	Qualitative Description
1st Class	70% +	Outstanding work which fully meets all criteria. Articular, logical presentation, with critical analysis, and substantiated and well-reasoned approach. Relevant use of material and clear understanding of research.
Upper 2nd	60–69%	Very good work with criteria met. Good use of resources. Evidence of discussion with justification of points made. Care shown with presentation.
Lower 2nd	50–59%	Good with most criteria met. Relevant material indicating understanding. Attempts at discussion, though some areas not fully covered.
Third	40–49%	Past standard – although work is limited in content, it satisfies basic criteria. Indication of understanding in the selection and use of material. Superficial discussion.
Fail	0–39%	Poor standard of work, meeting few criteria. Insufficient indication of understanding.

Fig. 12.1

work. This means identifying what those issues are and how the knowledge available in higher education can be used to increase understanding of them.

This raises a central tension for professional courses within higher education as they are never able to achieve the degree of detachment from everyday issues associated with traditional academic disciplines. Each course that awards a professional qualification as well as an academic award must demonstrate that at a minimum they produce practitioners who have acquired the skills and knowledge necessary for safe practice. Within higher education this sets up a tension between traditional academic courses where absolute control, by academics, over the curriculum is taken for granted and professional courses where the curriculum is subject to scrutiny by representatives of professional organisations. In many cases these representatives may not be academics themselves, but they will have the power to determine not only the content of the course, but also its length and structure.

INTEGRATING THEORY AND PRACTICE

It is clear from the above discussion that within the traditions of higher education it is customary for the lecturer to retain firm control over both the content and boundaries of the subject being taught. Any claims to student-centred education rest on providing students with the opportunity to identify difficulties and develop ideas, through dialogue with the lecturer, as the course is being taught. However, if we return to the work of Benner and Wrubel (1989), and of Schon (1983), it is apparent that they are concerned to identify the experiential knowledge gained by practitioners during the course of practice which, as discussed in Chapter Two, is qualitatively different from knowledge derived using technical rationality.

Similarly Eraut (1985) has argued that continuing or post-registration professional education should be concerned not only with imparting knowledge but 'should aim to enhance the knowledge creation and utilisation capacities of individual professionals and professional communities in general' (Eraut 1985: p.119). By this he means that professional education should concentrate on enabling practitioners to uncover the tacit knowledge implicit in their everyday practice. For instance, post-registration students are confronted with numerous complex problems during the course of their work which cannot be resolved through an appeal to technical knowledge. The elderly incontinent patient who refuses a bath, or the ill, depressed patient who refuses to get out of bed, are problems which nursing practitioners face regularly and for which there are no immediate or obvious solutions.

As discussed in Chapter Two, problems such as these rarely emerge as research problems, partly because they are viewed as 'basic' care which, it is frequently assumed, requires no skill or knowledge to implement. Such problems are not confined to nursing. Eraut (1985) has described a similar absence of knowledge to inform everyday activities in teaching. He goes so far as to argue that, 'in some professions nearly all new practice is both invented and developed in the field, with the role of academics being confined to that of dissemination, evaluation and post-hoc construction of theoretical rationales' (Eraut 1985: p.129). For Eraut, therefore, uncovering the knowledge implicit in practice means identifying knowledge that is generated by practitioners 'solving' individual cases and problems and identifying how this contributes to the practitioners' personal store of experience. Currently in nursing such knowledge remains private, is rarely published or widely disseminated. Subsequently it is unavailable to others who might benefit from it.

The wealth of knowledge implicitly developed by practitioners, offers, Eraut argues, a case for suggesting that professional education should provide a focus which enables practitioners to become aware of the tacit knowledge they are using and the valuable contribution it makes to practice. Such an approach truly does step outside the traditional boundaries of higher education to fully embrace student-centred learning in that it recognises the student as being in a position to define both the parameters and content of learning. Indeed the students are in a position to go even further and actually create that knowledge during the course of their practice and studies. This development clearly raises a number of issues for education not least of which is the need to distinguish between reflective education as it is developed for pre-registration students and reflective education for qualified practitioners. Secondly it raises a distinctive problem for assessment as, if the student is instrumental in identifying the content and the parameters of the knowledge base, then the criteria for failing discussed above can no longer apply.

ASSESSING REFLECTIVE LEARNING

The development of reflective education is very much a process of encouraging critical thinking on experiential learning. A variety of different teaching and learning strategies have been discussed in this book including the use of critical incident technique and learning diaries and the clinical studies assignment. Such methods are becoming increasingly popular in nurse education and are frequently seen as the hallmark of a reflective curriculum. The assessment of such strategies, however, remains contentious and problematic.

Assessing self-reflection

It is possible to argue that the movement away from technical rationality in nurse education has given rise to a particularly prominent interpretation of reflective learning which derives from the literature on psychology, communication skills and self-awareness. This interpretation appears to make a connection between a nurse's ability to analyse his or her own behaviour and motivations and the ability to reflect on practice issues. It is an interpretation that is grounded in many ways on introspection and a psychodynamic view of self. It suggests that, to reflect on practice, nurses first need to develop their ability to reflect on their own concerns, emotional responses, desires and motivations and to be able publicly to disclose these to peers and colleagues for critical review. Such an approach therefore uses the students' ability to reflect on themselves as practitioners, as a proxy for assessing reflective learning and by default reflective practice.

Teaching for self-reflection involves, therefore, developing strategies and techniques in which students are given the opportunity to disclose their emotional response to events they have witnessed or taken part in. This allows them to explore the taken for granted assumptions, values, norms, beliefs and ideas they might hold, which might determine how they feel about and, therefore, how they respond to a given situation. An example of this might be allowing students to discuss how they feel about men crying. These events can be practice-based or arise out of experiential learning situations such as role play exercises.

The development of such teaching strategies presents a central problem for nurse educationalists – namely the introduction of the 'I' perspective (for example, 'I was worried about this because . . .' 'I was afraid . . .' 'This made me feel very happy'). This is a particular problem if attempts are made to assess reflective learning through a self-reflection assignment. Traditionally the use of the term 'I' in assignments in higher education has been frowned upon as giving an account that is too subjective and partisan. If reflective learning is equated with self-reflection, however, the way a person feels – his or her emotional response to a situation – may be thought crucial as it determines subsequent practice behaviour. It may, therefore, form a central aspect of the assignment.

The problem with introducing the notion of 'I' or concern is that it can't be disputed or judged. While at an intellectual level it might be possible to argue that a student was right or wrong to be worried, afraid or happy, at an individual level this is an account of how the student felt at the time and is connected to the way he or she behaved. It provides a crucial insight into the student's behaviour and cannot be denied.

Attempts to promote reflective learning using self-reflection techniques such as learning diaries and critical incident technique recognises the importance of uncovering the meaning the situation had for the student concerned. The problem lies in how the student expresses this. Does the expression of this type of knowledge necessarily conform to the conventional essay style and structure? What do we do if someone chooses to write a story or make a confession, or if the work reflects the student's feelings of confusion or emotional turmoil about the situation and therefore confuses the reader?

Where students are asked to write up the process of self-reflection for the purposes of assessment they are frequently asked to supplement their descriptions of practice with appropriate references. Indeed this is true of both the clinical studies assignment and the learning diaries described in Chapters Ten and Eleven. However, in doing this we appear to be setting up a very artificial situation. In reality most of us perform our jobs on a daily basis without referencing each of our activities. Indeed many of us would be hard pressed to put an exact reference to how or when we learnt the knowledge which underpins many of our tasks and decisions. In reality we use knowledge from a variety of sources to complete work. These sources include experience, protocol within the department and an awareness of the strengths and foibles of our colleagues, all of which are crucial in determining not just what we do, but how we feel about what we do. By asking students to reference their daily activities we are, by sleight of hand, implying in no uncertain terms, that academic knowledge is superior to all other forms of knowledge in explaining practice. By default, therefore, we retreat back into technical rationality.

It would appear that the act of referencing reflective learning assignments transforms them into something artificial. Here students are asked to explain an aspect of their practice using respectable nursing texts, regardless of whether the texts make any contribution to understanding the situation described. The act of referencing could, therefore, re-construct the account according to orthodoxies of the literature rather than the student's experience. If the account given by the student is a construction then it no longer mirrors or 'reflects' reality, therefore one must question its links with reflective practice.

The strength of asking students to reference reflective practice assignments is that it allows assessors to judge the account given by the student in conventional academic terms, because following the traditions of higher education the process of referencing has objectified reality. While acceptable within the framework of higher education, this appears to defeat the learning experience in that it undermines the status of tacit knowledge while reinforcing the importance of abstract academic knowledge.

Interestingly, in our experience, most students are able to operate at both levels. They appear able to learn at a self-reflective, psychodynamic or affective level while accepting and conforming to an intellectual or cognitive assessment strategy. Indeed, their own taken-for-granted assumptions about education leads them to expect this. It would appear that, for most students, exercises like keeping a reflective diary are in themselves valuable learning strategies that are effective because students are so flexible in their ability to operate at a number of different levels simultaneously. This is supported by the very positive evaluation this type of learning strategy usually receives from students.

The major problem with developing self-reflection assignments, as with all assessments, is at the pass/fail borderline. In our experience most students appear able to learn at a personal and affective level while at the same time accepting the constraints placed on their freedom of expression by conventional academic language. There will always however, be some students for whom this remains a problem. Such students remain true to the purpose of the assessment, and to the guidelines given, presenting their work with all its raw emotional edge. Their account reflects the reality of their experience, but appears totally anecdotal, partisan and perhaps sensationalist to the reader. This type of assignment may have a high level of experiential honesty and emotional content. It fails however to connect the experience with the literature. This too may be intellectually honest as having read the literature the student may be unable to identify how it relates to their very personal experience. What they present is the truth as they see it and for this they fail.

They fail because in conventional academic terms it is difficult to mark personal accounts. An account can only be marked in-so-far as it conforms to academic definitions of what constitutes a good, analytical, well referenced piece of work. To the students, however, the result seems unreasonable as they were not asked to undertake a conventional assignment in the first place. Instead they were given guidelines which asked them to disclose their very personal and private experiences and responses to situations. When they do this honestly and refuse to play the academic game by introducing references which they consider spurious, they fail.

An alternative scenario is the student who loses all sense of the experience from which the assignment derives. In this situation the assignment may be of a very high academic standard using traditional higher education criteria, but fails because of its level of abstraction from any notion of experiential practice.

Both situations highlight the particular difficulties of setting and marking this type of assignment. They indicate the need to provide a very carefully thought out structure and set of guidelines for the student. They also highlight the need for a policy, to be decided before the assignment is set, which indicates that the above problems have been understood and strategies developed for dealing with them.

Under these circumstances the development of sensitive marking criteria is crucial to the integrity of the assignment. If the criteria are not clearly thought through it is all too easy to fail students because they display 'negative attitudes' or appear 'defensive', or because they fail to be critical enough of practice, which may in many cases be their own. This only compounds still further the students problems and is likely to ensure that next time the student will not be so naive as to be honest in their approach to the assignment. Examples of this type of marking include, for instance, assessing students communication skills according to a check-list of good and bad communication behaviour. The student may describe a difficult situation in which communication was poor. To fail the student on the basis of the account given does not acknowledge the difficulties they were dealing with or the student's courage in presenting the problem in the first place. Failure of this student is not an academic assessment but a moral judgement which fails people because they are not the 'right type of person', although what is the 'right type' is a matter of personal judgement which can quickly deteriorate into prejudice.

Such an approach echoes earlier debates in nursing, discussed in Chapter One, when nursing was seeking to establish its respectability as an occupation for middle class women. This is no longer tenable in today's society. The above analysis highlights how seemingly progressive educational developments can rapidly deteriorate into coercive strategies which serve only to reinforce historical ideologies and received morality in nursing.

It would appear that the arguments against marking, on a pass/fail continuum, self-reflective assignments are, therefore, very strong, particularly as the danger of using moral judgements about a person's 'worthiness' to do the course can so easily be disguised as criteria for passing or failing a reflective practice assignment. For this reason we do not assess the critical incident technique described in Chapter Nine. The learning diaries described in Chapter Eleven are structured in such away as to avoid discussion of the nurses' emotional or personal response to situations and instead students are encouraged to use academic language when writing them. This does, however, raise some problems for students and these are discussed in Chapter Eleven. Moreover, for additional safety, the diary is used as part of the formative assessment schedule and is not marked in the sense of passing or failing.

Both the critical incident technique and the learning diary do, however, form an important part of the course, although we recognise that by not formally assessing them, we may appear to be devaluing them. However at the moment we prefer to err on the side of safety and to proceed with caution. We hope that as our experience in this area grows and we learn more about these approaches we may tentatively be able to introduce a more formalised marking scheme. But as yet we do not feel we have the necessary knowledge, insight, sensitivity and ability to promote the type of honesty we are looking for in the essentially judgemental environment of an assessment.

Reflection as an intellectual activity

The above discussion of reflective learning derives primarily from a psychodynamic definition of reflective learning, which focuses on promoting self, reflection among students using a process of self-disclosure and analysis. It is possible to argue that, while worthy, such an approach is limited because it appears to focus exclusively on the individual and his or her problem solving and coping abilities. It tends, therefore, to promote the idea that individuals on their own can solve all the practice problems that they encounter. Failure to solve a problem or cope with a situation reflects badly on the nurse in question and indicates an inadequacy on his or her part. This again has distinct moral overtones.

It also tends to focus almost exclusively on inter-personal skills and nurse/patient interaction. While this is important it does not provide all the answers to every situation and indeed some situations demand very different solutions. However, if reflective learning is equated with self-reflection such solutions may not even be recognised or acknowledged. Occasionally very innovative solutions are condemned because the nurse did not solve the problem at the interpersonal level, choosing instead an environmental or resource strategy. However, this is not the only definition of reflective practice that is available to us. Schon (1983) provides quite a different approach when he discusses reflection-in-action. Here he talks about the need for experienced practitioners to articulate in an expressive way the myriad dimensions of their practice. He does not limit this articulation by artificial subject boundaries. He does not, therefore, suggest that reflective practice can only address issues at an inter-personal level, though such a level will obviously be crucial within nursing.Instead knowledge and its usefulness are defined by the practitioner who can draw on a variety of sources and solve problems at a variety of different levels. Therefore reflection might include consideration of the off-duty, or of supplies, hospital procedures or the impact of Government policies on practice.

Codes of conduct, ethical debates, accountability, multidisciplinary team-work and professional debates may all be relevant and, each on their own or in combination, may form a framework for thinking through a particular problem. They might guide practice, constrain practice or open up new approaches to practice unleashing new possibilities that were not avail-able under earlier scenarios. Making links between disparate develop-ments and identifying how they relate to everyday aspects of practice is crucial if nurses are to see themselves as part of a broader organi-sation and recognise their power to affect developments within this organisation.

Such an approach depends on the ability of the practitioner not only to recognise these links, but to be able to articulate their meaning and relevance for practice. In many ways it reflects the approach we have taken in the clinical studies assignment discussed in Chapter Ten. How-ever, it is difficult to see how such an approach could be used with pre-registration nurses particularly in the early stages of training. Using such an approach demands both extensive and intensive knowledge of practice. Student nurses, in the early stages of training, simply do not have this and therefore cannot be expected to undertake this level of analysis.

Reflective practice, as defined by Schon (1987), Benner (1984) and Eraut (1985) requires, therefore, as a pre-requisite substantive post-registration professional experience as well as a solid foundation of knowledge in the supporting disciplines. According to the above writers, reflective practice is characterised by a discussion of how knowledge is used to inform practice problems. The work of these writers implies that a reflective practice assignment would be similarly characterised by how well the students configured the knowledge from disparate academic disciplines, as well as from their own experience, to illuminate dimensions of practice. It is, therefore, a very high level skill which requires students judiciously to select only those aspects of a supporting discipline that are relevant to a practice problem and to integrate them in a way that reflects both the integrity of the supporting discipline and the specific dimensions of the practice problem.

To illustrate this the example of sudden death in an intensive care unit can be used. Here a student could discuss a massive array of literature. However, within practice two issues are likely to dominate the interaction between the nurse and the suddenly bereaved relatives. One is the issue of viewing the body. In a society where death and dying are hidden and institutionalised for many people this may be the first time they have seen a dead body. This will have to be managed alongside the issue of personal grief. The second is the issue of organ donation which is becoming increas-ingly important as surgical techniques improve. A traditional assignment in higher education, true to the positivist traditions from which it derives, might suggest the students should focus their essay on one or other of these major topics as it is not possible to do justice to both issues within the confines of a conventional essay. Not so lucky the intensive care nurse who has to negotiate both within a relatively short period of time, much shorter than it actually takes to write an essay and, in the case of sudden death, without any preparation.

This illustrates that students need first to undertake assignments on topics using conventional higher education approaches so that they can become knowledgable about each of the supporting disciplines. A reflective practice assignment, however, must assume this level of knowledge and allow the nurse to rehearse the dimensions of the problem as it arises in practice in all its messy complexity. The assignment could then focus on identifying the difficulties the nurses might encounter and possible strategies they could use to deal with these problems. The assignment could also consider what to do if the nursing strategies adopted go wrong. In fact the nurse might need to discuss how he or she would know if the strategy being used had gone wrong and what indicators could be used to recognise that discussions of an issue such as organ donation were unlikely to produce the desired outcome.

The development of an assignment that enables the student to rehearse the different dimensions of the problem is unlikely to conform to a traditional academic essay. There is, therefore, a need to consider the range of different structures that might facilitate this type of assignment. Students might narrate a story or give a case study or they could present the assignment as a discourse or annotated dialogue. They might present their material in the form of a diagram, map or flow-chart depicting the various possible directions open to the nurse at different points during the encounter. For instance, they could discuss whether it is better to broach the subject of organ donation before during or after the relatives had viewed the body. This could include a discussion of how they would know which was better or whether it made any difference at all. They could also discuss how some people might respond better if the topic of organ donation is introduced early on in the conversation, while for others a later introduction might be more appropriate. They could indicate how they would know which type of person they were dealing with. Such an assignment is unlikely to conform to the traditional format of academic assignments. It could appear quite unstructured and messy to the reader and may not draw on much literature.

Applying traditional marking criteria to this type of assignment would therefore, be inappropriate and could actually prevent its development. It is possible to suggest that if such assignments are going to be developed, then in a sense they need to be piloted first. Lecturers involved in education need first to try them out to see how they work and to appreciate both the problems of writing and marking this type of assignment.

Schon gives an example of this type of analysis when he discusses how professional sportsman such as tennis players can use this approach to improve their performance. He suggests that experienced coaches will use expressions which 'capture the complexity of action in metaphor ("lean into the slope") that helps to convey the feel for the performance' (Schon 1983: p.279). He suggests that, even within the fast pace of a professional tennis match, tennis players will practice for their performance by analysing small fragments of it in detail, such as placing the ball. The split second they have to act on this in the course of the match will be used to better effect if they have thought through beforehand the most advantageous approach to positioning the ball.

But again this is a rehearsal for the match. Tennis players are rarely judged on their performance during practice sessions, and so by implication it is again difficult to assess someone who is rehearsing for a performance and trying on for size the different approaches they could take to practice.

If the analogy is continued it recognises that all professional education is simply a rehearsal for practice and not an end in itself. Assessment should, therefore, be of practice and not of the rehearsal, as for the tennis player who is assessed on skills shown during a match and not a practice session. This brings us back to the central issue of this book, the links between education and practice. For the reasons outlined particularly in Chapter Two and elsewhere in the book, higher education has systematically downgraded professional practice as a lower order skill and emphasised the status attached to intellectual learning. Consequently we know very little that is constructive about the links between learning and practice. As yet we have few, criteria for assessing practice beyond a pass/fail dichotomy. In acknowledging this it is perhaps important to recognise that in pursuing reflective practice as an educational strategy we must be aware of our very limited knowledge base, of the fact that very few examples or exemplars of this type of learning are available to students and therefore we cannot expect them to solve issues we have ourselves only dimly addressed.

CONCLUSION

This chapter has outlined three different approaches to assessment; focusing on knowledge, focusing on self-reflection, or focusing on intellectual reflection. None of these approaches seem to offer a way to identify or reward reflective practice, indeed they may punish it. A reflective practitioner may not use knowledge in the accepted academic way; their practice may be unorthodox, and their attitudes may not be the 'right' ones.

The implications go further than simply failing to recognise reflective practice. Assessments which do not use appropriate criteria give those being assessed a sense of inadequacy if they are reflective practitioners, and a sense of complacency if they are not. Neither of these two outcomes is desirable, which suggests the need for a new type of assessment which not only integrates the different aspects of practice but which challenges the traditional criteria of current assessment. This issue is taken up in the next chapter which links the debates highlighted in this chapter with the enduring problem of assessing clinical practice.

REFERENCES

Benner, P. (1984) *From Novice to Expert: Excellence and Power in Clinical Nursing Practice*. Addison Wesley, California.
Benner, P. & Wrubel, J. (1989) *The Primacy of Caring Stress and Coping in Health and Illness*. Addison-Wesley, California.

Eraut, M. (1985) Knowledge creation and knowledge use in professional contexts. *Studies in Higher Education, Vol. 10, No. 2.*

Schon, D.A. (1983) *The Reflective Practitioner.* Temple Smith, London.

Schon, D.A. (1987) *Educating the Reflective Practitioner.* Jossey–Bass, California.

13 Assessment of reflective practice

Jan Reed and Susan Procter

INTRODUCTION

The previous chapter has discussed some of the problems of assessing reflection in written work. It has described these problems as arising from the lack of criteria we have developed so far, and in addition makes the point that what is mainly assessed in nurse education is rehearsal for practice, rather than practice itself. These two issues are the most crucial facing nurse education, and this chapter explores them further, focusing on the issues surrounding the assessment of practice. This is a somewhat artificial way of tackling the debate on assessment, for it separates thought and practice in a manner which is contrary to the principles of reflective practice. It does, however, reflect the existing assessment methods and strategies that we have at our disposal.

The problems of identifying criteria for assessing practice are difficult even if all that is required is a safe/unsafe result. The assessment must distinguish between acceptable and unacceptable levels of error, a distinction which is often difficult to make. The problems of identifying reflective practice, or advanced levels of practice, the issue currently facing nursing, is even more complex. What is needed is some way of distinguishing performance beyond the competent, if the aim is to recognise practitioners who are knowledgeable, skilled, effective, and creative in their practice.

If assessments are written or oral the problems of assessment are to some extent reduced, given that there are some guidelines available. These assessments, however, constitute reports or accounts of practice, and not necessarily practice itself, and so there is an argument to suggest that a valid assessment must involve some form of observation by the assessor. This is logistically difficult to do, given the time and resources available, but it is also difficult for a number of other reasons concerning the nature of nursing work. Nursing is a complex activity, with much hidden from the observer, and it also involves and is affected by the actions of other staff and organisational structures. These factors mean that the two most frequently proposed strategies for determining the level of nursing practice, task based and outcome based, are of limited value. This chapter discusses the problems of these two approaches, and concludes with an outline of a strategy that may be more appropriate to the needs of nursing.

TASK BASED ASSESSMENT

One way which has been used in many types of work is to grade practice according to the level of task that the assessee can perform. Thus different activities are graded according to the skill required to perform them, and practitioners can gradually work their way up the scale. Thus in carpentry, for example, a novice will be given very simple tasks initially, and will gradually move on to more complex work. Any assessment strategy will be based upon satisfactory performance of tasks set. This strategy is not as simple in nursing, however, because there is no clear agreement on any hierarchy of skills.

On first examination this statement sounds nonsensical, as most individuals will feel that they have developed such a model, and that their colleagues also share it. Furthermore distinctions are frequently made in nursing research, policy documents, and curricula, using terms such as basic nursing skills and advanced techniques. These hierarchies, however, are usually based on assumptions about physical care, and technological knowledge, assumptions which are increasingly challenged by notions of humanistic care. Such models might designate tasks such as bed bathing or feeding patients, as basic care, whereas reading monitors or catheterising patients are judged to be advanced techniques. There is some justification for this differentiation, as it can be argued that tasks in the former category represent fairly simple tasks, easily acquired, and which pose little threat to patients if incorrectly performed. The tasks in the 'advanced' category, however, are regarded as more complex, and more crucial to the survival of the patient.

The notion of increasing complexity, however, does not stand up to close examination. A bed bath is a much more complicated activity than reading a monitor, especially if complexity is judged as the degree to which practice can be adapted to individual needs. A bed bath has to accommodate differences in patient preference, health status, and clinical condition, whereas reading a monitor, or catheterisation is a fairly standardised procedure. Even if tasks are defined as competency in carrying out the stages of the nursing process (assessment, planning, implementation, and evaluation), it is difficult to arrange these in order of increasing complexity, as it is arguable that the knowledge and skills required for each stage are very similar.

The notion of impact on patient survival is also dubious. While giving a bed bath, the nurse could potentially cause great harm to a patient, equal to that potentially caused by incorrect catheterisation. Implementation of a care plan is no less risky or complex than writing a care plan. Other 'basic' tasks are potentially disastrous, for example giving an injection incorrectly in the buttock can paralyse a patient's leg if the sciatic nerve is damaged, yet this is considered a suitable task for first year student nurses. This point can also be made if we look at the tasks which have been passed on to nurses by doctors. At one time measuring blood pressure was considered so vital and complex a task that only doctors did it, whereas now it is part of the nurse's repertoire. Similarly tasks such as taking blood samples, suturing wounds, and giving intravenous drugs are becoming more common in nursing. The tasks have not changed greatly, and their import is not reduced, but now they can be delegated to nurses.

This suggests that the position of a task within a hierarchy of skill has more to do with how the task is viewed rather that the mechanics of its performance. The way that a task is viewed may have more to do with its mundaneness or status than with its inherent complexity or importance. This brings us back to issues about the status of nursing work, discussed in Chapter Two. Are we more likely to devalue work which can be classified as 'normal' women's work, and elevate technological care in order to preserve our distinction from lay carers?

Notions of humanistic care add another set of questions. The discussion above is conducted mainly on the premise that physical functioning is the most important part of health, and that health work is definable as a series of tasks. If this premise is challenged, as holistic and humanistic nursing challenge it, then the argument for a skills hierarchy becomes even more weak. If care is holistic, then it follows that it cannot be regarded as a set of tasks, but as a process which is viewed and evaluated as a whole. This is particularly the case where assessment is related to stages of the nursing process, as this strategy tends to fragment and compartmentalise care in a way which undermines the notion of integrated and concurrent nursing activity. If added to this, there is the notion that nurses give holistic care through some system of patient allocation, then it is clear that the care of any one patient can involve interventions of different types, and therefore the allocated nurse must be able to nurse in a number of ways and at a number of levels.

If we also acknowledge the importance of psychological and social factors in health, as well as the physical, then the picture becomes even more muddied. Nursing intervention in these areas is not so easily identified or demarcated as technical performance, especially if this type of activity is seen as an integrated part of nursing, underpinning and indivisible from giving physical care. Thus a bed bath becomes an action which maintains the comfort, self- esteem, individuality and personhood of the patient, rather than a simple exercise in hygiene. Dealing with technology, therefore, is not necessarily an advanced skill, and some would even say that this type of activity is a waste of nursing skills.

Another aspect of care which nurses are beginning to address is the organisational aspect. Nurses not only have to care for patients, but they do so within an organisational framework which determines much of their practice. It therefore seems logical that competence in this area could be used to differentiate between basic and advanced practice. With this framework, higher levels of practice could be characterised by communication, co-ordination, and management skills. Both the current UKCC and ENB proposals for establishing awards for higher or advanced practice appear to reflect this idea (ENB 1990; UKCC 1990).

This assessment focus can be described as looking at the organisational functioning of nurses, rather than the direct giving of nursing care. Characteristics such as 'changing practice' and 'communicating with other professionals' suggest a move towards looking at how nurses operate within health care organisations, and at their managerial skills. In many ways this can be seen as a step forward for nursing, in that assessing these abilities emphasises their significance in a way that has not been done before. It moves nursing skills into the domain of organisational issues, and thus highlights this domain as a legitimate one for nurses to become involved in. This may change nurses' views of themselves as victims of organisations to one of participants in organisations.

This strategy for defining expertise is a timely one, as health services become more and more dominated by management theory and values, rather than the traditional altruistic and humanitarian aims of health care. In order that these aims are not totally submerged by concerns about cost-effectiveness, there is a need for health care professionals to have an active role in the decision making processes of management, and this can be most effectively done by developing a greater understanding of organisational dynamics.

This may be politically desirable for nursing, and also justifiable when it is realised how much of nursing work is determined by organisational factors. It does, however, still pose problems for assessment. The question of attribution is problematic, in that managerial skills are by definition those which involve the behaviour of others, and nurses are still in a relatively powerless position in health care services. The degree to which a nurse can demonstrate skills such as changing practice, is largely dependent upon the permission given to nurses to do these things, rather than on the qualities of nurses themselves. There is still therefore a tension between regarding skill as the property of an individual (the basis of individual assessment) and viewing nursing activities as socially or organisationally determined.

Furthermore assessing these skills takes the assessment away from looking at that which is uniquely nursing. Management skills can be demonstrated by other professions, and so this form of assessment is not directly related to the giving of nursing care. Although there is a recognition that the work that nurses do for patients is not necessarily hands on care, to not assess this type of care seems to devalue it. Again there is a danger that direct caring skills will be seen as unimportant or taken for granted. Regarding organisational functioning as more advanced than giving hands on care could perpetuate this devaluation.

In short, nursing is more than the sum of its parts, and so we cannot assess nursing simply by looking at the activities nurses do, without looking at how these are managed, co-ordinated, and evaluated. Moreover nursing activities are frequently multi-layered, in that a simple procedure can also involve complex teaching and counselling, or can involve many difficult decisions. Developing a hierarchy of skills as a foundation for assessment is therefore an oversimplification of nursing work.

OUTCOME BASED ASSESSMENT

The complexities of nursing skill outlined above are problematic for assessment, in that they suggest no clear guidelines for evaluating performance in terms of the type of activity performed. Even if a hierarchy could be developed, simple performance would not necessarily solve all of our problems, because we would then need to look at the level of performance. What would be the difference between, say, giving a bed bath competently, and giving a bed bath well? The answer could be sought by one of two strategies. Firstly the behaviour could be examined as a discrete event, with attention focused on manual or interpersonal competence. This is problematic, because we cannot ensure that the assessed event will provide opportunities for the assessee to demonstrate the full range of skills that he or she possesses. A routine or straightforward activity will not provide opportunities for demonstrating that the assessee can think creatively, or adapt care to individual patients, or to deal with unforseen events. These are qualities which may well be worth noting if we want to identify levels of practice beyond simple competence. Secondly, this strategy is insufficient, because it fragments care, and does not relate the observed behaviour to the rest of the patient's experience, and if we wish to examine a nurse's grasp of the overall planning, implementation, and evaluation of care, such a 'snapshot' will not portray this.

This suggests a second approach to assessing performance; looking at nursing outcomes. Here the level of care given could be assessed by looking at the totality of the patient's care, and the result of that care. This, however, presumes that there is a simple causal relationship between care and outcome, but also that outcome can be attributed to an individual nurse. Given the individual nature of and response to health problems, the first assumption is dubious, and given the nature of nursing work, the second is also questionable.

The way in which nursing is organised means that the question of attribution is a difficult one. In most fields of nursing, care is given by a team of staff, especially if care is provided for 24 hours each day, over a period of time. As nurses only work 37½ hours per week, this means that patient care is provided by a number of staff, all working different shifts. Not all of these staff are qualified nurses, which means that some care must be delegated to students or to auxiliaries. In these circumstances care outcomes can only be attributed to the team, rather than to individual members.

This team working has been a cause for concern in nursing for some time. It has been seen as reducing continuity of care, and encouraging depersonalisation, and to address this nursing has developed several strategies. One of these is the nursing process, which facilitates continuity of care if not of carer, as there is an explicit system of planning care. This care may be given and evaluated by others, but the care planner is usually identifiable. Another strategy is the development of primary nursing, in which the nursing process is more formalised. Staff are identified as primary nurses for specific patients, and charged with the responsibility of planning and evaluating care. This system still does not ensure that the primary nurse will actually give the care, as this is a physical impossibility, but it is hoped that it will make clearer the accountability of nurses.

With these systems, the question of attribution becomes less difficult, but it is still not completely resolved. This is because there are also other health workers who have an impact on patient care, for example doctors, physiotherapists, occupational therapists and social workers. None of these workers can function alone; they are all mutually dependant on each other, and the outcome of care is largely determined by the degree to which their efforts are co-ordinated.

Assessing nurses by examining the outcomes of their care is therefore difficult, given the collaborative nature of nursing work. This collaboration is appropriate for dealing with the complexities of patient care, and also appropriate for staff development, in that it allows staff to contribute to decision making in ways that a rigid hierarchical structure could not accommodate. Attempts to change the way in which nurses work, for example by implementing primary nursing, may make the question of attribution less problematic, but these strategies, in effect, impose a hierarchical structure on to a system which has been collaborative. This may benefit the primary nurse, but not necessarily others in the team.

In addition to these issues, which are largely to do with questions about definitions of nursing, and the proper role of the nurse, there are likely to be methodological problems. No matter what the focus of an assessment is, whether it is on tasks or outcomes, there still remains a problem of how to gather valid information which will enable the assessor to evaluate activity. These methodological issues concern problems such as linking observable behaviour with unobservable thinking, in other words dealing with the problem of the right things being done for the wrong reasons.

ASSESSMENT METHODOLOGY

Assessment methodologies can be divided, at the risk of oversimplification, into two basic types. One is the written or oral assessment of knowledge or cognition, and the other is the observation of behaviour. As we mentioned at the beginning of this chapter, the written or oral assessment is useful for establishing the assessees ability to give coherent accounts of practice, but it does not allow us to look at practice directly. To do this we need some form of observational technique, and the discussion so far has been on what might be the focus of such observation. Observation, however, is also limited – not only can it observe inappropriate things, but it is possible that the analysis of observational data can be misinterpreted.

Using observation in assessment gives data on actual behaviour at the time of assessment. To argue from this data, however, that the behaviour observed is based on a sound rationale is stretching the data too far, and so all that this approach can do is ascertain that at the time of assessment the performance was broadly within approved procedures for practice. The observation schedule can be developed to enable the assessor to record and evaluate deviations from approved practice, and can even be developed to rank deviations as minor or major (rather like the faults system in horse jumping), yet in itself it cannot tell the assessor why these deviations occurred. What is missing from the data is any examination of the rationale underpinning behaviour, and this is a serious omission. Not only is it possible for people to do the right (approved) things for the wrong reasons, but it is also possible for people to do the wrong things for the right reasons.

To illustrate this problem, let us take the example of two nurses performing a similar task, changing a dressing, on two different patients. The first nurse may, to the observer, perform the task perfectly. This does not necessarily say a great deal about her knowledge or understanding of the principles of wound healing, it may only indicate that she has learned to do this task, in these circumstances. In a situation where something untoward happens, the nurse may not be able to reason from first principles to adapt her technique successfully. The second nurse may commit a number of procedural errors. She may do this, however, because the circumstances of the patient are such that she takes an informed decision to sacrifice some aspects of safety in favour of others, which she reasons are more important. This may involve having the patient in a position awkward for the nurse, but comfortable for the patient, using unorthodox instruments, or applying the dressing as quickly as possible because relatives are outside, waiting to say goodbye before they leave for holiday. The first nurse passes the assessment, the second nurse fails.

The injustice of this result is only evident because these illustrations contain some description of the processes of thought which have determined the behaviour of the nurses. Without this information the result would seem fair and sensible. Assessment by simple observation, therefore, does not really tell us much about abilities, which suggests that we need a more interactive and integrated form of assessment, one which studies both thought and action.

This methodological problem has long been recognised in research, and has led to the development of methodologies which may have something to offer assessment techniques. One example is the ethogenic approach pioneered by Harré and Secord (1972) which combines observation with discussion of the events observed. The purpose of this discussion is to uncover the rationales and perspectives which the actor uses to explain his or her actions. The researcher will therefore ask the research subject why he or she did certain things, what other things could have been done, and what were subject's aims in doing what he or she did. This type of information makes it possible to link behaviour to thought, avoiding the often banal explanations people often give of their actions in the absence of observed examples. Asking people to describe their work without reference to examples often results in the production of 'glittering generalities' which provide little illumination of the way in which they behave.

A similar approach was used by Benner (1984) in her research. Here she observed nurses, and also used accounts of practice as springboards for discussion. These discussions were firmly anchored to real-life events, preventing them from drifting off into abstract realms of conjecture and generalisation.

These approaches, using data about practice as material for discussion, have something to offer nurse assessment, in that they seem to bridge the gap between thought and action. Assessment, however, is a very different situation from research, and this will affect the use of these strategies.

Assessment is primarily a judgemental exercise, in which the assessor must judge whether the assessee has passed or failed according to pre-determined criteria. Research does not have this responsibility or these constraints, its task is to describe phenomena, analyse them, and communicate this analysis. If researchers start to judge data in terms of acceptability, they would be quite rightly criticised for having a biased approach. It is therefore easier for a researcher to obtain 'unlaundered' accounts of practice from people than it is for assessors, whose role is interpreted by the assessee as looking for the 'right' answers.

This adds a stronger element of self-justification to the assessee's account. Moreover, this self-justification is couched in what are thought to be acceptable terms for the assessor. This raises two important points about assessment methodology. Firstly there are questions about what are the 'right' answers, or acceptable rationales for assessment, and secondly there is the problem created by having these criteria and the way that they determine the assessee's response.

Taking the issue of 'right' answers first, it can be seen that this is problematic. The first section of this chapter discussed the different ways in which the concept of advanced practice could be viewed, and identified some of the problems associated with each view. This section simply looked at the complexities of nursing work which make expertise so difficult to pin down, and it did not attempt to explore different approaches in any great detail. What was clear from this discussion, however, was that nursing is an activity determined by individual patients' needs and organisational factors, all interacting in complicated ways which are possibly unique to every different situation and event. How then could nursing assessment hope to distinguish between right and wrong rationales in these circumstances?

Clearly what is needed is not a system of right and wrong, but a system of valid and invalid answers. This validity has to be essentially contextual validity, in other word the assessor needs to ask 'Does this account make sense in its own terms, for this particular situation?' rather than 'Is this the right way to go about things, according to my criteria?'

This position takes the view that if the assessees can justify actions adequately, then their account will be accepted. This offers the opportunity to tap into the assessees' knowledge of their particular context, and their particular patients. If, for example, the assessor asks why a nurse did not contact a patient's family when planning a discharge, the nurse could reply that this was not done (in defiance of hospital policy) because the patient had pleaded with staff not to inform relatives, or because the district nurse had felt that it was better for her to contact them, as she knew them well. These rationales may well be considered valid by the assessor.

This approach has the virtue of recognising the uniqueness of practice, and avoiding over reliance on decontextualised regulations about what is a 'good' rationale, but it does skirt dangerously close to an 'anything goes' position, which is not really what is wanted. In the face of a strongly argued rationale, the assessor must have some guidelines for distinguishing between sound and unsound explanations of practice. The work of Schon is helpful here, in that this work does map out reflective processes and patterns which lead to successful resolution of problems. For example Schon talks about 'framing problems', the process of trying out different frameworks to see which one fits the problem best. Using this idea, assessors could seek to discover if this process has been undergone, asking the assessee what alternative approaches were considered. The final choice of approach is ultimately idiosyncratic, and difficult to challenge, but the assessor's concern would be that the assessee had considered a number of other approaches.

Criteria like this may provide a useful framework for identifying advanced practice, but as yet this work is in its infancy and not yet developed enough to allow universal or uncritical adoption. Even when such criteria are more fully developed, operationalising them may be by no means a simple matter. Using this type of framework involves changing assessors ideas about assessment, but also assessees. This brings us to the second point about assessment, the expectation held by the assessee that there are 'right' answers.

This raises the problem of self-validation, an inherent characteristic of professional work, as Friedson (1971) argues, which means that professionals are often adept at denying inadequacies or problems in practice, because they cannot afford to admit to them. Holden (1990) also argues that the stress of professional practice, particularly in medicine and nursing, leads practitioners to search for certainty in their work because uncertainty is difficult to deal with. They therefore search for logical explanations for events, and construct coherent accounts whether these actually match their actions or not.

This problem of self-validation occurs in research and assessment, but it is particularly tenacious in assessment, due to the judgemental nature of this activity. The pressure to concoct a rationale for behaviour in an assessment is very strong, and it is likely that this concoction will largely be determined by the culture of nursing and of assessment. If the culture of nursing is seen as intolerant of deviations from orthodoxy, and assessment is seen as an exercise in identifying these deviations, then assessees who are skilled at presentation will camouflage their activities under the current professional rhetoric, and those less skilled (or more honest) will approach the assessment with fear and dread. In both cases the assessment will not reflect anything more than the ability to articulate practice in the currently ideologically acceptable way.

CONCLUSION

The debates outlined above suggest two things. Firstly they suggest that we cannot assess practice in a meaningful way without some kind of dialogue between the assessor and the assessee. Without this dialogue we are in danger of making unfounded assumptions about the abilities of nurses, because we do not examine the thought processes which underpin their actions. Secondly this chapter suggests that even if we have this dialogue, our problems will not necessarily be over, because if this is seen as an inquisition, looking for orthodoxy, then the accounts nurses give of their practice will be tailored to what they think we want to hear. This problem is also compounded by the fact that we do not know what we want to hear.

This conclusion suggests that assessing practice is an insoluble problem. This is not necessarily so, but what is certainly needed at the moment is a period of reflection within the profession. We need to know more about what we are looking for when we talk about expertise, and so we need to explore these issues further in research and education. We need to think more about the implications of our decisions, and be prepared to regard them as temporary rather than final. We need to amend and develop approaches in the light of thoughtful evaluation and debate.

   This debate is a daunting prospect, as what we, as educationalists, find difficult to cope with is uncertainty. In much the same way as nurse practitioners, we too seek self validation. This debate would, however, be a productive one, if only because it would openly acknowledge doubt, freeing nurse education from the pressure to know all the answers.

   This has implications beyond assessment, for assessment is inextricably linked to educational process. If we are open about assessment, we must therefore be more open about education, otherwise we will face contradictions between the way we teach and what we see as the purpose of this teaching. This openness may allow us to move from knowledge transmission to facilitating knowledge creation, as Eraut (1985) suggests. We could then begin to listen to our students more carefully, to help them in the process of articulating their knowledge, and ultimately learning from them. With a clearer picture of the issues practitioners face, and the ways in which they face them, we could provide education tailored to their needs, whether this be basic knowledge or reflective exercises.

   In some ways this process has already begun, with the work of Benner and Schon which has allowed us to listen to practitioners and acknowledge the legitimacy of their accounts. Their stories were success stories, an important point, as previously practitioner knowledge had been viewed as inadequate or incomplete. Perhaps what we need to do now is to look at the failure stories, the problems that practitioners feel that they cannot solve, and to look at these in a non-judgemental way. In order to do this we need to create a climate in nursing in which nurses can admit to failure without fear of reprisal or censure, and creating this climate in our education system is perhaps the first step.

REFERENCES

Benner, P. (1984) *From Novice to Expert: Excellence and Power in Clinical Nursing Practice*. Addison Wesley, California.

English National Board for Nursing, Midwifery and Health Visiting. (1990) *Framework for Continuing Professional Education and Training for Nurses, Midwives and Health isitors*. ENB, London.

Eraut, M. (1985) Knowledge creation and knowledge use in professional contexts. *Studies in Higher Education*, Vol 10, No: 2. 117–133.

Friedson, E. (1971) *Profession of Medicine: A Study of the Sociology of Applied knowledge. Dodd Mead*.

Harre, R. and Secord, P.F.(1972) *The Explanation of Social Behaviour*. Basil Blackwell, Oxford.

Holden, R. (1990) Models, muddles, and medicine. *International Journal of Nursing Studies*, **27(3)**, 223–234.

Schon, D. (1983) *The Reflective Practitioner*. Temple Smith, London.

United Kingdom Central Council for Nursing, Midwifery and Health Visiting. (1990) *The Report of the Post-Registration Education and Practice Project (PREPP)*. UKCC, London.

14 Future developments in nurse education

Jan Reed and Susan Procter

INTRODUCTION

The problems of coaching and assessing reflective practice are, as the previous chapters have pointed out, extremely difficult, given the nature of nursing and the constraints that this places on nurse education. The problems discussed in previous chapters have been at a micro level, in other words at the level of the teacher, the student, and the course. In this chapter we turn to the macro level, in other words the development of national frameworks for nurse education, and look at reflective practice in light of recent proposals from professional bodies, in particular the proposals for post-registration education developed by the UKCC (1990) and the ENB (1990).

Recent developments in nurse education can be summed up as demonstrating a move away from knowing facts towards knowing how to learn. Knowing how to learn, it is argued, is a more useful approach to take in a profession which has to deal with changing health care systems, changing health care needs, and changing health care knowledge. Perhaps the most crucial step that nursing took towards this model was the development of Project 2000, with its emphasis on independent learning, and developing the skills of analysis and critique in student nurses. The Project 2000 curriculum comes close to notions of reflective practice, albeit only in a somewhat tentative way, but it is envisaged that the type of practitioner which will qualify from these courses will be in many ways different to previous cohorts of newly-qualified nurses.

What the nursing profession is now turning its gaze towards is post-registration education. This is entirely logical, as to have a situation where a nurse undergoes a dynamic and creative initial education programme, and then stops at the moment of qualification, is to do an injustice to practitioners. Not only will the skills of learning that they have developed become rusty, but any thirst for learning that they have will be frustrated. In addition to this, a basic training programme, however independent the learners it produces, is unlikely to prepare them fully for the potential changes in health care throughout their career, especially if their career allows them little time or support for study. For those who have undergone pre-Project 2000 training (and they will be the majority of nurses for some time to come) the situation is even more bleak. Not only do they have to cope with meeting new ideas without the skills of Project 2000 nurses, but they also have to mentor these nurses, assess them, and ultimately compete with them for jobs. Furthermore, as Eraut (1985) argues, 'The quality of initial professional education depends to a considerable degree on the quality of practice: and that in turn is influenced by the continuing education of the practitioners.' (Eraut 1985: p. 131.) These are powerful arguments for the development of some kind of framework for the continuing education of qualified nurses.

There are some additional arguments to be made in favour of the re-organisation of post-registration education. One of these is the argument that nursing deserves greater academic recognition. When basic nursing courses were not recognised academically, and post-registration courses offered little more, the opportunities for nurses to develop through these courses were limited. When nursing was not interested in academic credibility this was not seen as a major problem. Academic credibility is an issue for nursing now, perhaps as part of the striving for professional status, perhaps because nursing has become more confident about its knowledge. The introduction of Project 2000 courses at Diploma level can be seen as an illustration of this concern. This still, however, leaves the basic level of nurse education at a level lower than many other professions, at a time when graduate status is being sought by many comparable occupational groups.

Another set of arguments for changes in post-registration education are related to the current organisational changes in the NHS. As health services do become more cost-conscious, and nurses are managed more and more by people with little health care or nursing experience, the question of nursing skills becomes crucial. As the employment of non-nurses (who are after all, cheap to train and employ) gains pace, a coherent argument in favour of the qualified nurse is vital. As the activities of nurses and non-nurses can appear to be very similar to the outsider, there needs to be a way of making the benefits of employing experienced qualified nurses more apparent. A system of post-registration education which clearly identifies experienced nurses and the roles that they can fill is one way of asserting the value of employing such nurses.

This is the venture that nursing is embarking on at the present time. It is a difficult one, as we have no history of describing or assessing clinical work apart from distinguishing between safe and unsafe practice. It is not surprising then, that the initial ideas about how this can be done are linked very closely with concepts from academic models. Whether this link can be made, and whether ideas about intellectual development can equate with the development of practice knowledge are fundamental questions which need to be debated. It may be that academic and practical skills are two very different animals, and they cannot be integrated into one all-embracing framework, or it may be that our ideas of academia and of practice need to change. What is clear, however, is that the professional bodies responsible for nursing are concerned about post-registration development, and are attempting to develop mechanisms by which nurses can be recognised for their expertise. The success of this project, however, is determined not only by theoretical considerations, but also by the degree to which it addresses the issues that practitioners face in their clinical practice.

CURRENT DEVELOPMENTS IN CLINICAL PRACTICE

The proposals for changes in post-registration education will not, in themselves, revolutionise nursing unless the expertise that they reward and foster is also rewarded and fostered by an appropriate career structure. Differentiation between levels of practice will remain no more than a paper exercise unless it can be translated into different clinical roles. This is beginning to happen to a limited extent in nursing practice, and in fact pre-dates the educational proposals, but progress has been slow and uneven. Part of the reason for this lack of progress may be, conversely, that the educational framework has not been in place to support such career developments, for appointing nurses to different clinical positions has been an arbitrary and confusing process. Without a framework which indicates different levels of practice managers have few clear criteria for making appointments.

One example is the recent clinical regrading exercise. This exercise was an attempt to recognise different levels of practice, and to link them to different practice roles and different salaries. Instead of nurses simply receiving automatic increments based on length of service in their post, nurses can now move from grade to grade. This exercise has had considerable teething problems which would appear to arise from a lack of consensus about how the characteristics of each grade should be interpreted. As they are based on job descriptions which seem to assume clear boundaries for the work nurses do, it is not surprising that this has happened. As much of nursing involves teamwork, and involves 24 hour care from staff who only work up to 37½ hours per week each, it is obvious that nurses must be prepared to perform duties outside their own job description, if ward organisation and patient care is not to suffer.

This blurring and sharing of roles is essential if nursing care is to be coherent, but it poses a problem of defining levels of practice in terms of specific duties. It also puts nurses in a difficult position when negotiating with managers, because they may very well reason that it is just as effective to appoint staff at the lowest grade possible, as they will perform the duties of higher grades when necessary.

Another problem with the regrading exercise is that it is not tied to any framework of qualification or assessment. Some advertisements for jobs are requesting particular courses for particular grades, but this is not universal or standardised throughout the health service. It is therefore unclear what qualities and skills each grade demands, and how these can be demonstrated or assessed.

There are, however, other developments in the organisation of nursing work which may go some way towards resolving these issues. Firstly there has been for several years now, an increasing number of clinical nurse specialists. These nurses have specific areas of expertise, and are available on a consultative basis to staff within their place of employment. They are not usually tied to wards, and can therefore focus on a very clearly defined type of nursing input, usually giving advice and information to staff and patients. This role is one which fits quite easily into grading structures – the job is clearly defined, and specific qualifications can be identified.

The proportion of nurses having these roles is, however, limited. What patients also need is nurses who will give a range of care when necessary, rather than only specialised inputs. This daily care is, arguably, a rich field for developing expertise, for it is crucial care. The scenario of this care being given by a range of specialists, however, is horrific. For patients to be bathed by the bath specialist, to have their temperature taken by the observation specialist, and their interaction conducted with the communication specialist, all of whom are moving from ward to ward, is a state of affairs which will clearly lead to fragmentation of care, and is equivalent to the task oriented nursing from which we have tried to escape. Nurse specialism is therefore a limited option for defining expertise.

Secondly, primary nursing may be an alternative strategy for defining and recognising levels of nursing practice. Here nurses take responsibility for the total care of small groups of patients, and manage and organise members of the team that they work with. Decisions are taken by the primary nurse who plans care, and evaluates care when given. This is very similar to the role of the traditional ward sister, but instead of the ward being organised as a whole it is divided into smaller units, each unit having a primary nurse, (or mini-sister) in charge. This scheme potentially offers the opportunity for nurses to develop their skills of planning and managing and as such could provide a way of identifying levels of practice.

This system has been tried in a relatively small number of nursing units and, so far, has not been fully evaluated. The evidence there is suggests that nurses have greater job satisfaction if they are primary nurses, but patient response and care outcomes have not yet been investigated in many units. What does seem likely, however, is that logistic problems will begin to emerge, again due to the nature of nursing work. The primary nurse will work only for a fraction of the hours that a patient needs care, and so there will obviously need to be some delegation of responsibility to others, who may be unqualified. This creates the problem of role blurring and sharing mentioned earlier.

If the 'official' primary nurses are to be qualified nurses, then this may result in increased financial costs for health care organisations. The numbers of qualified nurses per unit may have to be increased to ensure that teams are adequately supervised and care monitored. One strategy which may be used to overcome this is to increase the number of patients that each primary nurse is responsible for until the new system can be accommodated within existing staff provision. There comes a point, however, where the whole purpose of primary nursing (to give personal and individualised care) is lost as these numbers of patients increase. In a thirty-bedded ward it can be seen that primary nursing is realisable with, for example, five primary nurses each caring for six patients. If this is financially expensive, and managers opt for a system of, say, two primary nurses responsible for fifteen patients each, then this is starting to look more like simple task allocation under a new name. Another strategy would be to use unqualified staff as primary nurses, but this strategy again blurs the distinction between levels of practice.

If primary nursing is adopted and financed adequately, however, it will provide a demonstration of different levels of nursing skill. Team members could be regarded as those who can follow instructions competently, whereas primary nurses would be those with sufficient knowledge to plan, modify, and evaluate care. This does, however, run the risk of fragmenting care, and dividing staff into those who plan care and those who give care. (This not only begins to sound like task allocation, but it also creates an artificial distinction between tasks. Assessing, planning, and evaluating are activities which are concurrent with implementation, not separate from it). The measure of these abilities would be ultimately in the outcome of care, with 'good' primary nurses being more 'successful' than 'poor' primary nurses. This of course raises important issues about what is successful in nursing, and also questions about what sort of educational support primary nurses will need to be successful. A knowledge of health care problems and nursing procedures will not necessarily be enough. This knowledge will eventually be out of date, and so primary nurses will need to be able to update their knowledge, but they will also require additional skills in management, organisation, planning and problem solving.

These skills were largely the province of the ward sister who made decisions which other nurses then carried out. The ward sister has traditionally had very little preparation for this role, but this has not mattered so much in the past when nursing simply followed the instructions of medical staff. Now when nurses are required to make nursing decisions, they cannot simply follow orders, and so must have an adequate basis for decision making.

These developments in the way that nurses are working, and roles that they are taking on, offer possible ways of distinguishing between levels of practice. They are matched by developments in the way that post-registration education and development is beginning to be discussed. These educational developments are also concerned with updating knowledge and with differentiating between levels of practice, and it is to these initiatives that we turn now.

PLANS FOR POST-REGISTRATION EDUCATION

At present there are two schemes in British nursing which are receiving great publicity. These are the schemes proposed by the UKCC for post registration education and practice (PREPP), which discusses a level of practice called 'The Advanced Practitioner', and the English National Board scheme which offers a framework for what they call 'The Higher Award' (UKCC 1990; ENB 1990). Both schemes are broadly similar, and at the time of writing it is unclear as to how they will be put into operation, so the following discussion will be devoted to the principle which underpin these ideas, rather than the details of the schemes.

Both schemes share certain ideas, namely that there should be a formalised way of recognising expertise, and that this way should be linked to Higher Education, more specifically to the Credit Accumulation and Transfer Scheme (known to most people as CATS) developed by CNAA (the Council for National Academic Awards). It would probably be useful therefore to look at CATS in greater detail before looking at the issues that arise from this linkage.

Credit Accumulation and Transfer Scheme (CATS) is a scheme developed under the auspices of CNAA for use in Polytechnics and other colleges of Further and Higher Education. It is largely a response to the perceived need to make Higher Education more flexible and easier to access. Growing demand from mature students without traditional 'A'-level qualifications, and students who may wish to take breaks from education, move to different courses, or to different institutions, required a system which would accommodate these students in some coherent way. There always has been an informal system by which Higher Education could meet these needs, but it was idiosyncratic, depending on the policies of individual course leaders and different institutions.

From this very brief description, it can be seen that CATS was developed for use within mainstream Higher Education, for academic courses. This can also be seen from it's basic unit of analysis, the three year undergraduate degree, which is used as a framework to rate courses. In the CAT scheme the three year honours degree is seen as consisting of;

Year One	120 level one CAT points
Year Two	120 level two CAT points
Year Three	120 level three CAT points

Thus students who have completed part of a course have accumulated CAT points which can be used towards another course if they wish. It is based upon ideas of progression in academic ability throughout the learning career, and therefore students must collect points at each level before they can move onto the next. This process is made more meaningful if the courses are organised in modules, so that students can accumulate CATS points as they work through the course, rather than gaining them at the end of each academic year.

The CAT scheme does not allow students to pick and choose freely; it demands some connection between the modules studied. It is unlikely therefore, that someone could, for example, do some history, some engineering, and then apply to join the final year of a Fine Art degree, unless they could convince the CATS panel, who would examine their case, that these subjects were related, and that the level one and two points gained would equip them to study art at level three.

As part of the CATS remit, a system of developing alternative routes for entry into courses is also being developed. These schemes are known by the acronyms APL (Accreditation of Prior Learning) and APEL (Accreditation of Prior Experiential Learning). APL is possibly the easier of the two, as it will examine courses studied. These will hopefully have clearly defined content, some indication of academic level, and a form of assessment. In recent years, the CNAA has accredited many ENB courses, which has made a significant contribution to facilitating access to HE courses for many nurses. APEL is a much more difficult exercise, as it will include a vast array of learning experiences which may have not been assessed or evaluated, and may be very individual. An example would be one of the courses that nurses attend, the Open University package, 'a systematic approach to nursing' (ENB 553). Those who have attended this course will know that some people worked hard on it, learnt a lot, and it changed their practice. Others were not interested, did very little work, and forgot the course as soon as it finished. It would clearly be unfair, therefore, to give equal credit to all participants, but without some form of assessment there is no way of distinguishing between those who learned from the course, and those who did not.

APEL can include attendance-only courses, conferences and study days, and also work experience. Again experience is difficult to equate with learning. We can all think of nurses with 20 years of experience in the same job, who know very little about their work, nurse in the same way as they did when they began, and are regarded as a liability in the ward team. We can probably think of others who have got to grips with their job, studied to learn more about it, and became excellent, dynamic, and creative practitioners, within a very short period. Clearly the number of years service does not necessarily say anything about a person's experience or knowledge. In order to come to some conclusion about a person's ability then, it is obvious that each individual case must be examined carefully.

This is possibly the most crucial issue for CATS – the extent to which this process is feasible given the financial and resource constraints of higher education. If each individual student who wishes to use CATS needs a panel to examine his or her case, which may require an interview, or even some written work assessed, then the system can only cope with small numbers of students. This process might become more straightforward if a systematic way of dealing with APL and APEL is developed, but at the time of writing this development work is at a very early stage. Even with this system in place, the input required from higher education will be far more than for the traditional student with 'A'-levels, who wishes to do one course, and whose application can be dealt with by one admissions tutor in the space of five minutes.

There is however, a clear wish on the part of higher education to increase access and flexibility. This has led to the development of special access courses, such as the Higher Education Foundation Certificate (HEFC) and an increasing interest in distance learning. The progress of these developments, however, will depend much on adequate resources and finance. At present each full-time student attracts funds from local education authorities (LEA) and higher education funding bodies. The resources coming into the institution are therefore considerable, which enables the institution to pay for staff, heating, electricity, teaching materials, and accommodation. There is, however, very little surplus in the system, and non-traditional students, who might not bring equal funding with them may have to be subsidised by traditional students. An example is a part-time student on a nursing diploma or degree course, who is judged to be equivalent to a fraction of a full-time student in terms of funding. This student may require a level of teaching and supervision which is very close to, if not more than, a full-time student, but attracts less than half the funding. A student who joins a course for some modules, who is using the CATS system, may not attract any funding at all apart from his or her fees. As student fees are usually low in comparison to costs, then such students may only be a viable financial proposition if their fees are increased. It is unlikely that these will be paid by LEAs or health authorities, and so students may have to meet this burden themselves. Neither the ENB nor the UKCC have given clear guidelines on how the advanced awards are to be financed, and it is unlikely that the new Higher Education Funding Council, which will manage funding in all Higher Education institutions, will be making provision for an unknown number of nurses to be supported in HE.

These are some of the financial and pragmatic problems facing higher education at the moment. They may be resolved, but it is unlikely that there will be a massive increase in funding to cope with these initiatives. For nursing to link up with higher education is, therefore, not a simple matter financially. Someone will have to pay for any services that higher education provides, and there is a strong possibility that this may be the individual nurse who wishes to take part in any professional development scheme. This situation is further complicated by the possible integration of Colleges of Nursing and HE within the next few years, which could further increase the difference between pre- and post-registration education and access.

There are also some theoretical issues involved. As mentioned earlier in this chapter, CATS is based on the three year degree academic course structure, and this gives rise to a number of problems if it is to accommodate professional development. In order to discuss this more fully, we need to look at these professional development schemes more closely.

PREPP and the Higher Award

Both of these schemes outline some notions of levels of practice that nurses can aspire to. These levels of practice are largely pragmatic, in the sense that they involve different ways of functioning and behaving in the clinical area. This is eminently suited to the needs of the nursing profession, which is concerned not only with knowledge, but with performance.

This concern with performance is not, however, restricted to competence at specific tasks, it also involves a cognitive component. Higher level practice will not just consist of say, giving an injection better than a novice, but will involve an understanding of wider issues surrounding practice. This does run the risk of taking nurses away from the bedside, and into the realms of management, but this is perhaps a reflection of new emerging definitions of practice in nursing, that it does not just involve practical skills, but also involves an organisational role. The focus on these wider issues does actually make the task of identifying levels of practice easier in some ways, as assessment of cognitive abilities is easier than assessment of behaviour beyond a safe/unsafe classification.

What then will the advanced practitioner look like, and what qualities will this person have? Both the UKCC and ENB frameworks cover issues such as planning care, communicating with other professionals, decision making, and evaluation of care. Both frameworks also mention the ability to utilise research in care-giving, and the ability to teach patients and other staff, along with the ability to manage change in health care delivery. These characteristics are, arguably, a combination of behavioural and cognitive phenomena and as such are faint echoes of concepts of reflective practice. This is not explicitly mentioned, but the research on which the proposals were based, in particular Fish and Purr's (1991) project paper for the Higher Award, are informed by the concept of reflective practice. What is perhaps more clear is the vision expounded of the future practitioner as an independent learner, autonomous practitioner and active participant in the organisation of health care.

How then will a practitioner be able to demonstrate functioning at this level? This is a thorny question. Although the abilities or characteristics are couched in behavioural terms, both official bodies advocate that aspiring practitioners should undertake some form of educational programme, which implicitly recognises that these skills cannot be derived from practice alone. Completing these programmes however, cannot guarantee a level of practice commensurate with the criteria outlined above – assessment of knowledge does not always denote anything about practice.

There seems to be an expectation that a modular scheme, developed through CATS, will provide indications of functioning at a higher level. This is not necessarily the case. CATS is an academic scheme, based upon the acquisition of academic knowledge, and is largely concerned with facilitating and organising entry and progression in HE. The assessments that a CATS student undergoes are the responsibility of the teachers providing the modules that the students take, and not part of the CATS remit.

Furthermore, as mentioned earlier, CATS is based upon the structure of a three year undergraduate degree, a structure which involves prerequisite levels of achievement before students can progress. There is some suggestion that the Advanced Practitioner/Higher Award will be equivalent to 120 level three points, in other words the final year of a degree. This poses logistic problems in accommodating the many nurses who have no level two points, as CATS will not enable them to bypass this stage. This central notion of progression in CATS also poses a problem if a course leading to advanced practice has to be designed to cover all of the characteristics required at level three, without there being any coverage of these issues at lower levels. The assessment load is therefore likely to be high in this type of course, and will not necessarily match the traditional pinnacle of assessment on degree courses – the final year project or dissertation. This final assessment is much cherished in HE, as it allows students to study a topic in great depth and to demonstrate their skills in handling and organising material; indeed many of the previous assignments on degree course are rehearsals for this final hurdle. CATS, therefore, is not a mechanism that will ensure integration of theory and practice, in the way that the official bodies seem to expect.

The only way that this can be done is by close and careful collaboration with HE to develop specific modules and assessments which will meet these expectations. Again, however, this is problematic. HE can assess knowledge and understanding in written work, but it has not concerned itself to any great extent with assessing professional functioning, apart from the assessments it makes of undergraduate student nurses. HE can cope, therefore, with the cognitive components of any higher award, but this will not provide any evidence that the students is behaving any differently to other non-advanced practitioners.

Traditional nurse education may not be able to address this issue either, as discussed in the previous chapter. Here again, practical assessment has been concerned with basic safety, and the focus has been to observe students for limited periods of time, to satisfy the observer that the student is competent. Clearly, however, more than competence is required in these professional development schemes, and the skills which need to be identified are not amenable to brief observation.

This problem can be illustrated by looking at one of the characteristics identified in both schemes, the ability to change practice. An academic programme could concentrate on the student's knowledge of change theory, evaluation strategies, and organisational analysis, and could even go so far as to set assignments requiring students to discuss these theories in relation to their own practice. This would not mean that the student could operationalise this knowledge, it would simply indicate that there was an understanding of the concepts involved. It is difficult to see, however, how any clinically situated assessment could do more – is it possible to observe somebody changing practice without being with them for prolonged periods of time?

If, for the sake of argument, we assume unlimited resources, and some-one does observe a nurse throughout the process of changing practice, this still raises the question of attribution, in other words how much of the change can be attributed to the nurse in question. Changing practice can be facilitated or hindered by a number of things outside the nurse's control, for example health policies, financial decisions, or the views of other interested groups. The success of a change strategy does not, therefore, depend upon the nurse alone, who is often in a comparatively powerless role in the organisation.

Looking at the success of a change strategy, therefore, does not necessarily say anything about the change agent, and in addition poses problems of grading. Grading academic work is clearly defined in HE, but as has been mentioned before, is not established in practice assessments. Would it be possible to award grades for this ability? It could be argued that grading is not essential, and the focus is on whether a nurse can change practice or not, and it therefore does not matter whether a nurse passes narrowly or with flying colours. This, however, brings us back to the pass/fail classification of traditional practice assessment, which is contrary to the spirit of the proposals, in that they are seeking to move beyond the identification of basic competence.

The problem of grading practice also calls into question the ability of an academic CATS scheme to accommodate this type of assessment. The basic structure of point levels is based upon academic criteria, i.e. usually written work, with clear differences expected in work produced on courses at different levels. Whereas we are reasonably clear as to what we mean by level three written work, there is no consensus as to what constitutes level three practice, or how this can be distinguished from level two practice. The levels are not simply determined by the content of the assessment, but by the level of ability to deal with the content expected from the student. Therefore demonstrating characteristics is not enough, there must be some way of identifying the level to which these characteristics are being demonstrated.

There are therefore two dimensions to grading, the level that has been achieved, and the degree to which the level has been achieved. In other words students will not only pass a course at a particular level, but they will also be passed at different standards, ranging from the borderline Pass to, in the case of an Honours degree, First Class standard.

If these levels and standards cannot be accommodated within HE, then nursing may have to develop its own form of CATS. This would arguably be more appropriate for professional needs, but would not integrate nursing into higher education. It would remain marginalised and be regarded as faintly eccentric. This is not necessarily a problem for individual nurses, but professional bodies may well see this situation as a frustration of their ambitions. If the aim of the professional development proposals is to achieve academic recognition for nursing, with a corresponding professional status, then a separate system would not achieve these aims.

These problems and issues are exactly the same as those identified in the previous chapter, which concluded that the best solution may be some form of integrated assessment, in which both behaviour and knowledge are explored. This might be along the lines of various phenomenological or ethnographic research strategies, which seek to look at 'real life', and the participant's understanding of it. The assessment strategy would therefore resemble the research methodology of, say Benner (1984) or Schon (1983), with observation and discussion combined within the investigation.

This may be an appropriate theoretical solution, but it is not necessarily feasible. Anyone reading research studies of this type will appreciate the length of time involved, and the theoretical understanding required of the researcher. Their task, however, is comparatively straightforward compared to that of the educational assessor, as their concern has been only to describe and analyse specific phenomena, not to evaluate behaviour according to criteria of skill.

The problem is compounded by the fact that we have very little knowledge upon which to base these criteria, in other words knowledge about the hallmarks of expertise, how they are developed, or how they can be identified. The characteristics of expert practice identified in recent proposals are not substantiated in the proposals by any reference to research literature. We are therefore faced with the issues of whether these characteristics are empirically validated, and whether we know enough to distinguish and identify them. Without this exploration we may find ourselves unable to recognise the really important skills of nurses, and following some political agenda instead, which is all about what professional bodies want us to do, rather that what we actually do. Will we have reflective practice developed in a technical rationality mode?

CONCLUSION

The proposals for the development of post-registration education obviously have some problems. Firstly there is the issue of relevance to nursing careers, in other words, what's in it for the practitioner? Having expertise recognised may give nurses a glow of satisfaction, but if this is all it will give them then support for these schemes will be limited. This is, however, a 'chicken and egg' situation – an educational and a career structure are mutually dependant, and it is impossible to say which should come first. The importance of a career structure goes further than this, however, as it emphasises the value of the qualities necessary for career progression. This provides others with role models and exemplars, and sets the agenda for professional development. If reflective practice is to become the aspiration of nurses, it follows, then, that it needs to be organisationally as well as educationally rewarded and facilitated. Without this recognition, reflective practice will remain hidden and undervalued.

Secondly, there is the problem of linking professional development to an academically-derived structure. The shortcomings of academia have been debated in Chapter Two and Chapter Twelve, the conclusion being that academia cannot address practice issues unless it changes radically in they way knowledge is viewed and developed. If it does not, then post-registration schemes may involve no more than an academic 'rubber stamp', or, more dangerously, be reduced to academic exercises with no relevance to practice. Again, this is not conducive to the development of reflective practice.

Thirdly, there is the problem of assessment, and this is where the development of reflective practice is perhaps most at risk. Without a well thought out strategy for assessment, the 'expertise' being rewarded may be something quite different from reflective practice, and in addition, may discourage reflective practice. If the criteria of post-registration schemes are interpreted in a mechanistic way, with notions of 'right' and 'wrong' answers, or without questioning the issues of validity which arise from problems of attribution, or notions of a hierarchy of skills (see Chapter Thirteen), then a reflective practitioner may well be disadvantaged. The nurse who will pass with flying colours may well be the one with the skills to present favourably in light of current ideological fashion. Although these skills are valuable in some circumstances, they are not what reflective practice demands.

The proposals for developments in post-registration may turn out to be an opportunity for reflective practice to develop in nursing, or they may not. Much depends on how these changes are introduced and interpreted, a difficult operation given the size and diversity of the nursing profession. It is tempting, therefore, to present proposals in as simple a form as possible, without discussing the complexities and ambiguities of the principles which lie behind them. This certainly gives the initial impression of clarity, but does not help those who later find themselves becoming confused. Both the ENB and UKCC proposals run this risk, and in so doing run an even greater risk of having their intentions misinterpreted, and their objectives lost, as educationalists attempt to operationalise these schemes.

Reflective practice, therefore, is in a very vulnerable position at the moment (although, perhaps, no more than it has been in the past). Having begun to understand and describe reflection and expertise, we may extinguish these rare and tender plants by insensitive handling. This suggests, therefore, that we need a further period of thinking and debating before we zealously rush to promote what we do not yet fully understand.

Postcript

The incompleteness of our understanding of reflection and expertise is something that we and our colleagues are very aware of. What seemed simple ideas became increasingly problematic when we attempted to apply them to our teaching, and many of these problems are not resolved (and perhaps they may not be resolvable). We do feel, however, that we have made some progress, but this has been largely dependent upon the situation that we work in, which is characterised by strong peer support, interaction with teachers from other disciplines, a fair degree of personal autonomy, and encouragement (verging on exhortation!) to challenge received wisdom. Without these factors our interest in reflection and expertise would have remained casual, and it is unlikely that we would have attempted to integrate them into our teaching.

Because our interest was spontaneous, and implementation of these ideas was not enforced, we have developed our teaching at a leisurely pace. The discussions and teaching strategies in this book have had a period of development lasting for several years. We do not feel that this process can be enforced, or can occur in environments where orthodoxy is valued more than independent thought. It follows, therefore, that the greatest danger to the development of nurse education is that notions of reflective practice and expertise become the new orthodoxy, which is unchallenged and unchallengeable. This is not only premature, but it is contrary to the spirit of these ideas. In conclusion, therefore, we would argue that what nursing needs now is a period of reflection on reflective practice, and the opportunity to develop expert knowledge about expert practice.

REFERENCES

Benner, P. (1984) *From Novice to Expert: Excellence and Power in Clinical Nursing Practice*. Addison Wesley, California.

English National Board for Nursing, Midwifery and Health Visiting. (1990) *Framework for Continuing Professional Education and Training for Nurses, Midwives, and Health Visitors*. ENB, London.

Eraut, M. (1985) Knowledge creation and use in professional contexts. *Studies in Higher Education*, Vol 10, No. 2, 117–33.

Fish, D. and Purr, B. (1991) *An Evaluation of Practice Based Nursing in Continuing Education in Nursing, Midwifery, and Health Visiting*. ENB, London.

Schon, D. (1983) *The Reflective Practitioner*. Temple Smith, London.

United Kingdom Central Council for Nursing, Midwifery, and Health Visiting. (1990) *The Report of the Post-Registration Education and Practice Project (PREPP)*. UKCC, London.

Index